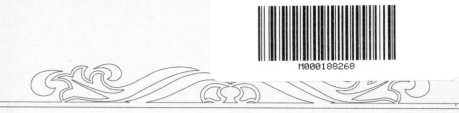

SOMETHING SPECTACULAR

The True Story of One Rockette's Battle with Bulimia

GRETA GLEISSNER

SEAL PRESS

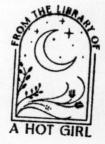

SOMETHING SPECTACULAR
The True Story of One Rockette's Battle with Bulimia

Copyright © 2012 by Greta Gleissner

Published by
Seal Press
A Member of the Perseus Books Group
1700 Fourth Street
Berkeley, California

Library of Congress Cataloging-in-Publication Data

Gleissner, Greta, 1973-
  Something spectacular : the true story of one Rockette's battle with bulimia / Greta Gleissner.
      p. cm.
  ISBN 978-1-58005-415-7
  1. Gleissner, Greta, 1973—Health. 2. Bulimia—Patients—United States—Biography. 3. Dancers—United States—Biography. 4. Women dancers—United States—Biography. 5. Rockettes (Dance company) I. Title.
  RC552.B84G54 2012
  616.85'2630092—dc23
  [B]
                                        2011045965

9 8 7 6 5 4 3 2 1

Cover and interior design by Domini Dragoone
Printed in the United States of America
Distributed by Publishers Group West

FOR GRANDMA PATTY AND GRANDMA SALLY

Contents

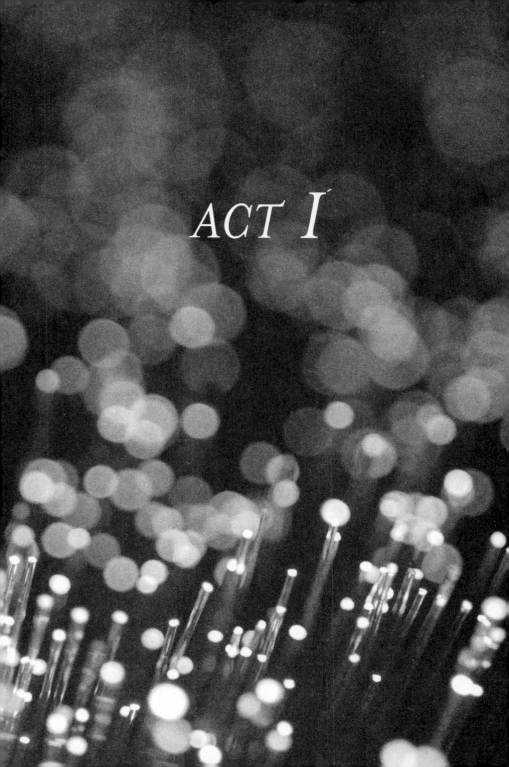

ACT I

Overture

I t's eleven in the morning and I'm already back. The familiar gush of wind from the air conditioner sweeps across my face and adds a little more frizz to my already curly mane as I pass through the automatic doors of the supermarket. The same cashiers are still diligently scanning products and punching in produce codes. Across the store, dressed in his white button-down shirt and paisley tie, the manager scurries about wearing the required ass-kissing smile of a customer service professional in New York's Upper East Side.

Although the customers are different than they were on my last visit, their faces are the same: contemplative stares as they squeeze cantaloupes and scrutinize apples, each vying for the perfect fruit; eyes filled with frustration and lips curtly positioned, as they steer their carts down doll-sized aisles. From aisle to aisle, I dart past these faces like a woman on a mission. My statement is clear. I know what I want. Don't try to get in my way.

As much as I frequent the D'Agostino's on Eighty-Third Street and Lexington Avenue, I should receive some sort of special recognition—food vouchers, for Christ's sake, or at least one of those boxes in the bakery with the bright orange sticker filled with day-old donuts. It doesn't take me long to gather the necessary items, as I have memorized the exact layout of every aisle. Standing in the checkout line, I'm hoping the checker doesn't notice that I've already been through her line once today. As a rule, I alternate checkout lines attempting to remain as anonymous as is possible for someone who enters the same grocery store day after day. Right now, however, I'm in a hurry and my impatience will not tolerate a long line.

I place my items on the revolving black belt in a deliberate manner, trying to give my high-caloric food choices an innocent facade. After looking at my selection of Hershey's Kisses, Reddi-Wip, sour cream, cheddar potato chips, French onion dip, cinnamon rolls, chocolate donuts, and a twelve-pack of Diet Coke, Emily S., as the label states on her nametag, which is almost covered by the "Five Years of Dedicated Service" sticker, becomes inquisitive.

"Are you having a party?" Emily S. asks.

This exact question has come up dozens of times by other prying cashiers, but my conscience still cringes with embarrassment every time.

"Yes, I am. It's my roommate's birthday."

The lies roll off my tongue so naturally. If she only knew the truth. Occasionally, I tell cashiers, "No, the food is for me," which sparks their curiosity and inevitably leads to a discussion of how lucky I am to be able to eat so much and stay so thin. For a moment, I gloat, telling each of them that my secret is my fast metabolism, which, of course, is another lie. Today I don't have time for idle chat. I need a fix.

Emily S. bags my items carefully, in her own style, at her own pace. Clearly, she's clueless about my sense-of-urgency. *You're not bagging eggs, Emily S., only binge food.* Just as I want to reach over the counter, grab this pimply-faced cashier by the neck, and tell her to hurry the fuck up, she smiles pleasantly and responds.

"Okay. Your total is $24.61."

Finally. I shove my ATM card in her direction, praying that I have enough funds in my account to cover the bill. While waiting for my card to process, I realize that Emily S. has failed to notice the twenty-ounce Diet Coke bottle sitting next to my purse in the grocery cart. I don't feel obliged to let her (or any of the other cashiers) know that she has failed to ring me up completely. I mentally rehearse my prepared story for the security guard who may tap me on my shoulder as I exit the store.

"But officer," I will say, "I thought that she saw my Diet Coke. Isn't it *her* responsibility to look in my cart? Sorry, I guess I wasn't paying attention."

This imagined exchange between some middle-aged, wannabe-cop security guard and me never takes place, but I am still nervous every time I leave the store, thinking about the undercover Diet Coke cop potentially waiting outside to arrest me.

Bags in hand, I head down Lexington Avenue to my next destination: Pick A Bagel. On the way to my favorite bagel shop, I can't help but notice the many undernourished stay-at-home mothers. Usually their nannies accompany them, pushing the kids in a stroller alongside. These women are so busy with personal trainers, personal shoppers, and decorating luxurious brownstones that they simply can't live without nannies. I'm jealous of these women, whose lives appear so picturesque. If only I could have what they have, then I would be happy.

In my heart, I know this is a lie. Beneath the forced smiles and conservative Chanel maquillage lie a misery and emptiness with which I deeply identify. There's a certain hollowness that doesn't discriminate based on social class.

Nonetheless, I still want what they have. Looking down at my frumpy self—Rockette sweatshirt, Broadway Dance Center cut-off sweats, which I've been sleeping in for two days, hair heaped on top of my head—I suddenly feel embarrassed. Haunted by hollowness or not, these mothers are ten years older than I am and look better than I ever will. I'm a mess.

Tomorrow, I will start to live my life differently.

Unable to wait to eat until I arrive at the Pick A Bagel, I break open the airtight bag of Hershey's Kisses. Chocolate aromatics race out of the bag as it bursts open, soothing my nerves. Unraveling their shiny aluminum jackets excites my mouth. My taste buds vividly recall the succulent bites of milk chocolate perfection. Chugging my stolen Diet Coke in between bites, I pop Hershey's into my mouth one kiss at a time to tide me over as I make my way to my next destination.

At Pick A Bagel, ten or more people are already in line. I want to scream. My body *is* screaming. It infuriates me to be waiting in line at a time like this. All I want is to walk into an establishment, buy my "drug" of choice, shove massive amounts of it down my throat, and then spew it out a couple dozen times, until I have reached my goal—pure numbness.

My anger is not only for the long line. I'm angry with myself for ending up here again. Like every other morning, I had promised myself that today would be a *good* day. A good day means eating perfectly—no bingeing, no purging, and eating three, low-fat meals. Once again, my day has turned into one of wasting money, wasting time, and wasting my life.

Scanning over the familiar array of cream cheeses, three different choices of tuna and chicken, made-to-order salads, and fresh-baked bagels, I engage in one of my favorite pastimes: planning my future diet. *Let's see . . . I will have a toasted "everything" bagel with butter for breakfast, a fat-free salad for lunch, and for dinner I can have . . . .*

"Are you ready, lady?" asks the man behind the counter.

Oh, sure. Now you want my order. Interrupt me as I'm planning my perfect diet, you rude asshole. Before answering, I force a smile in the direction of this man who insists on calling me "lady."

"Yes, may I please have two sesame bagels with egg salad and American cheese?" Five minutes later, my bagels are neatly wrapped and ready to go.

"$6.87, lady," he says with his hand held out, as if I've already wasted too much of his time.

"Here's $8," I say, throwing the money at him. "Keep the change."

I'm not quite ready to go home to Eighty-Third Street and First Avenue. One block away from my one-bedroom apartment is the best white pizza and greasiest crust that I've ever eaten. Pizza Man (he has no other name, as far as I know) gives me a familiar, friendly smile when I walk through the door. I'm a regular, ordering take-out pizza from him three to four times a week for a year now.

"How you doin'? May I help you?" Pizza Man asks.

Pizza Man likes to stir up conversations. Under other circumstances, perhaps when I'm not trying to emotionally and physically destroy myself, I wouldn't mind having a nice chat. But today, I come out of desperation.

"Can I get two slices of white pizza and two slices of pepperoni?" I ask Pizza Man. "You don't have to put them in the oven. I'm in a hurry."

After hiking up five flights of stairs, I'm finally inside my apartment. My bags and I go straight to my bedroom in case my roommate, Vivian, comes home. Vivian and I met in an Overeaters Anonymous meeting. She's also bulimic; the main difference between us is that she's in recovery. If Vivian knew what I was up to, she'd say that I was a threat to her recovery and I'd have to move out immediately. I don't care. I'll take my chances.

I constantly change my housing arrangements in an effort to escape my eating disorder—as if it's possible for me to escape from myself. No matter how many times I hear it, I fail to grasp that "recovery is an inside deal." Instead of digging down to the core of my authentic self—the self that so many of my past therapists attest that I have—I move from coast to coast, go in and out of treatment, and believe that I can externally act my way out of this addiction. The day I moved out of my Astoria apartment for the last time and hopped onto the N train heading toward Vivian's apartment in Manhattan, the excitement I felt was somewhat tainted by the truth. I knew how this story turned out. Moving to the city wasn't going to cure me.

The problem with having roommates when you're bulimic is that they're free to pop in and out of the house whenever they please, even if you've managed to memorize their schedule. Vivian is an actor. She's working today at Shakespeare in the Park in Central Park, so I should be safe, although there are no guarantees.

Now in my room, I can finally relax. Grabbing the remote, I flip through the channels until I find my favorite soap opera, *All My Children*. Still popping chocolate kisses into my mouth as I delve into the dramatic lives of Erica Kane and Adam Chandler, I spread my food out onto my bed. *Hmm. Which foods to eat first?* Carefully, I create the perfect food combination, attempting to maximize the satisfaction that the salty-sweet binge food will bring me. I keep plastic D'Agostino's bags close to my side just in case Vivian comes home from work early and I have to hide my binge food. I shove large bites of egg salad sandwich into my mouth first, alternating with handfuls of chips and dip. Delight absorbs my veins as I pack as much food as I can into my mouth without choking. My mind is a blank slate, forgetting any of the earlier remorse I felt about wasting my life. With each swallow, the creaminess of the egg salad and cheese sandwich coats my soul. Moving on from the first sandwich, I rip through the box of cinnamon rolls and release the protective seal on the Reddi-Wip. Large squirts of whip cream top each bite of cinnamon roll before penetrating my palate. After a few minutes, I have to take a break.

I've trained my stomach to reject any sense of fullness, so I have to take breaks in between food groups to throw up. I can't throw up in our shared bathroom, however, because Vivian could discover my secret. My only option is the plastic D'Agostino's bags. I really don't like to purge in plastic bags. Sometimes a bag has miniscule holes that I only discover once I see vomit dripping out of it. Moreover, there's a storage issue. When no one is home, I can easily throw the bags down the trash chute; but in the case that Vivian comes home right after I'm finished, then I have to store the bags in my closet and hope that the acid from the vomit doesn't split open the bags.

Besides the strategizing that I have to do daily, hourly, or some-times, minute-by-minute, purging has become very easy for me. I just lean over and out it comes, which is both a blessing and a curse.

My alarm clock reads 2:15 PM. Two hours have gone by and I'm forty-some dollars poorer. Yes, that's about the amount of time and money it takes to elevate my mind onto a plateau of pleas-ant paralysis with no thoughts or anxieties to fret about, just an opiate-like numbness induced from the rise and fall of my blood sugar. My body wants nothing more than to hide under my duvet and dream away the day, but I can't relax, yet. The magnetic tug of tiredness yanks at me as I stand up from my bed. I gather my bags and wrappers, walk outside of my apartment and traipse down the hallway to toss any evidence of my pathological behavior into the trash chute. Heading back toward my apartment, I can't help but feel regret for wasting another day. *You fat pig. You have no self-*

control. Back to my room I go, finally able to turn off the lights, close the curtains, pull the covers over my head, and act as if none of this has taken place.

In my mind though, I can't deny my actions. I don't understand why I can't discipline myself and eat the way that I want to. I hate myself for breaking my promises again.

There's always tomorrow. Yes, tomorrow will be a good day.

A couple of hours later, I hear the clanks of Vivian's keys, the turn of the brass doorknob, and the front door moaning for a lube job as it swings open and slams shut. For weeks now, I've noticed by the way Vivian escapes to the gym whenever I'm home, and by her suspicious glances when she eyes the amount of oatmeal, butter, and Equal in my morning breakfast bowl, that she may know that all is not what it seems in my world of recovery. I don't want to face her today.

I can hear her in the kitchen. Our apartment is a large one bedroom—which really means that we live in a six-hundred square-foot, including closet space, Upper East Side box—so I hear her every move. The opening of the refrigerator door, the hard jerk of the jammed silverware drawer, and the pop and peel of the aluminum seal on her yogurt container tells me that Vivian is making her abstinent afternoon snack.

The creaky hardwood floors chase Vivian's footsteps, as she wanders into the living room. I expect her footsteps to stop in their usual spot—in front of one of our Papasan chairs, the chairs we call our satellite dishes—but instead, the creaking grows louder as her footsteps near my bedroom.

I unleash my head from the despair dwelling under my covers and lunge my body over the side of the bed. Balancing with my arms, I maneuver my upper body into an upside down pushup position, cock my head sideways, and press my cheek as close to the floor as I can to glance underneath the crack of the door and see what's happening on the other side. My nose crinkles as microscopic particles of dust and cat dander fly into my nasal cavity with each inhale.

A shadow of feet appears underneath the door. *Don't knock. Please don't knock.* My eyes seal shut, as I silently repeat the mantra, hoping to send a shot of cosmic energy through the door to make Vivian turn away. I walk my hands in reverse up the side of my bed, until I'm sitting up straight again. I stare at the paint-chipped white door and wait. In case she feels inquisitive enough to knock, my mind fumbles through the possibilities of plausible excuses as to why I've condemned myself to my room. After a few moments, her shadow disappears, as if she no longer cares what I've been up to all day. Maybe she already knows.

Since I relapsed on my food four weeks ago, my bedroom door has been the great divide between my actual truth and the truth that I present whenever I'm in Vivian's presence. Several months back, I promised Vivian that if I relapsed I would first, tell her, and second, not binge and purge in the house. Now I've failed to do both. At the time that I moved in with Vivian, I had sixty-two days of abstinence—well, give or take the three or four purges that I chose to ignore because they were so minimal—so it seemed easy enough. However, like all of the other times I've tried to stay binge-purge free, I felt the eventual itch that every food addict experiences right before she (or he) says, "Fuck it!" and relapses.

I throw my white duvet back over my head. I'm depressed. Here I am, trapped underneath my comforter, all because I'm too afraid to face Vivian. I can't believe my life has been reduced to this. I'm twenty-eight years old and I'm hiding from my roommate because I can't knock my food addiction. With each breath I take, hot air rebounds from the duvet to my lips. This is why I've never been able to sleep with the covers over my head. I have a suffocation phobia. A lingering smell of vomit revolves in my space and taints the air each time I exhale, reminding me of my nasty behavior. It doesn't bother me. I've gotten used to smelling like puke.

I wonder how long I can stay in my room before Vivian will call the mental health authorities. Will she even notice? Maybe she'll be so mad at me for breaking our agreement that she'll leave me to rot under here forever. I'm paranoid. An annoying nag in my head keeps whispering to me, *Get up, Greta. Just get up.* I don't want to get up. I know that I'm going to have to face Vivian at some point. She may not suspect anything. *Greta, just get up. Fine, fine, fine, I'll get up.* Reluctantly, I slink off my bed toward my bedroom door and force myself to come out of my disease-infected room.

I open the door. Vivian's eyes are piercing mine. Uh-oh.

"Hi," I say, in my best I'm-so-surprised-to-see-you voice. "I didn't hear you come in."

Vivian sits on one of the satellite dishes and nervously twirls her blond hair. Her pale eyebrows frown at me with concern, as if they're about to ask me a serious question, but they refrain.

She cracks a hesitant smile. "How are you?"

I dart past Vivian barely making eye contact and grab my Diet Coke in the kitchen to avoid a possible interrogation, as though my carbonated beverage and evasion tactics will somehow shield me.

"Fine," I say. "I was just taking a nap. I think I may be coming down with something." It was a poor lie.

I take a big chug out of my Diet Coke as I walk back into the living room. *Ahh.* Artificially sweetened carbonation is my beer. It takes the edge off. I keep gulping out of my one-liter bottle, silently counting from one to ten, as it takes about ten counts of chugging before I feel like I've had an all-consuming satisfying swallow. As I near my last gulp, my eyes shift to Vivian—she's at it again—nail biting. Her fingers look beat up, with exposed nail beds and cuts around her cuticles from the constant gnawing, which, I have to say, is disgusting. Vivian's teeth have sawed her nails down so much lately that I didn't know there was a nail left on her ten fingers to chomp on.

"Greta," she begins. "We need to talk."

Shit. I think she knows. How can she know? I mean I haven't been *that* obvious. Maybe she doesn't know.

My mind zips in rewind to replay all of the snapshots of bulimic episodes I've engaged in over the last month, times when she could have noticed my behavior. I question my offensive behavior, as if I'm filling out the section on an employment application asking me to check yes or no about whether I've ever been convicted of a felony or misdemeanor. Question No. 1: Have I ever left food or bags of puke in my room for her to find? No. Question No. 2: Regarding the times I threw up in the toilet, did I ever leave a mess that she could see or smell? No. Question No. 3: Have I eaten any of her food? No.

I've covered my tracks. No need for further explanation. Anything she thinks she has on me is circumstantial, not enough evidence for a conviction. Still, an addict can smell relapse like a wild animal smells its prey.

Vivian rises from the chair and transitions into her proverbial pigeon-toed, insecure, hunched-shoulder stance that she settles into whenever she faces a confrontation. Her hands slide into the pockets of her denim overall shorts; shorts that hang sloppily over a white Gap T-shirt, a getup that went out in the early nineties. Her eyes hold a combination of fear and guilt, as if she's a twelve-year-old girl who has to tell her mother that she just broke her favorite earrings while playing dress-up.

Fuck. I recognize those eyes. I've been through this before with other roommates. The look in their eyes that precedes the conversation about how my insanity is tugging on the threads of their sanity, blah, blah, blah, and they can't deal with it anymore. I don't want to have this conversation. Not today.

"Greta, I . . . I know you're relapsing."

Vivian's words are barely louder than a whisper, but the meaning of them stuns my insides.

Me, relapse? Who's relapsing? I haven't been relapsing. My naturally manipulative instinct is to turn around to see what other bulimic in the room she's talking to, but I know there is no one else.

"I've known for weeks," she continues, her voice now gaining confidence. "I've been trying to ignore it, but I'm struggling to stay abstinent myself. I can't be around you. You're threatening my recovery."

Excuse me? I'm threatening her recovery? Like she hasn't been compulsively exercising and starving herself the entire time I've been living with her. Now I feel like a twelve-year-old.

I walk over to the couch and take a seat. A sobering moment such as this is too much to handle in an upright position.

"Are you saying that I have to move out?"

Out of the corner of my eye, I see Vivian's two cats, Osiris and Mambo, who sit tall on the window ledge, ears erect with intrigue. They, too, want to know.

She takes a deep breath, pulls one hand out of her pocket, and begins to twirl her hair again. The seconds become sluggish. Her focus is everywhere, on the bookshelf, on the coffee table, on the wall. Just not on me.

"Yeah, I guess that's what I'm saying," Vivian says, bravely.

After a few moments, her eyes have the courage to meet mine.

"You know I care about you." She looks at me as though she has no other choice. As if I have put her in an ethical dilemma. "I just can't have the behavior in my apartment."

You self-righteous, little . . . I start to get angry with her, but stop myself. I know where my anger lies.

My hands catch the weight of my head as it collapses with shame and regret into my palms. "I don't know what to say." *You stupid fucking bitch, what's wrong with you? You can never get it right. Why can't you just eat the way you're supposed to? You fucking idiot!* I had plenty of words for myself.

"Vivian, I'm sorry," I say, my tear-soaked hands muffling my voice. I meant it. I never wanted this to happen.

Vivian comes over to the couch and sits next to me. She's no longer my roommate. She's my friend again.

"I really wanted this to work. I just can't do it anymore. You can take a week or two to find an apartment. It's not like I'm going to throw you out without a place to go. I'm going to stay at my father's for a few weeks."

"Thanks, Vivian. I'm so sorry, really."

Kicking High

f I get this job, I'm going to change my life. I've said this at least a
dozen times throughout my life, when auditioning for dance schol-
arships or other dance jobs, but this time I'm serious. No more
bingeing and purging. I will plan my food, go to my Overeaters
Anonymous meetings, save my money, and live the way I've always
dreamed to live in this city. I mean, it really is just that simple. If I
become a Rockette in New York, then I will finally feel good enough.
Such an accomplishment will force my eating to improve. Success
breeds success, right? That's my hope; though I never seem to be able
to follow through.

I'm standing midblock on Fifty-First Street between Fifth and
Sixth Avenues outside the stage door entrance. There are more than
two hours to wait for the clock to strike 10 AM, before the plump—but
powerful—dwarf of a man standing guard by the door will hand me
my security badge to audition. I have nothing else to do but sit on the
sidewalk and watch the talented hopefuls filing in line behind me. As
they pass by, I can't help but snicker. Musical theatre dancers are all
the same. They show up all bubbly with their inflated charm, standing

in their pseudonatural, duck-like, look-at-me-I'm-a-dancer stances. They plant air kisses on the cheeks of fellow dancers and speak much too loudly about what auditions they've landed or what fabulous and amazing people they'll be working with later on in the week.

It's important to note that I'm one of these dancers. If you asked, I'd tell you just how much I love *Cats* and *42nd Street*. If you peeked through the window at Starbucks, you'd find me sitting at a table reading *Backstage,* planning what auditions I was going to attend the following week. The difference between me and the other dancers is that I'm the star of my own one-woman play. That is, I participate in the absurd grandiosity of the musical theatre world, pretending to live and breathe auditions, eager to land the next job. The truth is, however, I rarely go to auditions. I hate them. The only reason I can push myself to audition to become a Rockette is that I'm the perfect type: tall, leggy, with an extensive tap, jazz, and ballet background. And there isn't a singing requirement.

I don't have to be a psychologist to know that my hatred for other dancers stems from an overwhelming sense of inadequacy. It's jealousy, really. Not for their talent, I can hold my own in that department. It's because of the self-love that seeps from their pores as they speak, in all of their glorious animation, emitting sweet fragrances of crisp confidence and zeal. Other dancers don't skip auditions because they feel too fat or too ugly to attend. They don't skip class because they've spent all of their money on binge food and are too exhausted from puking all day. They don't sit in restaurants by themselves eating an appetizer, entrée, and dessert, while excusing themselves several times to go to the bathroom. They don't steal their roommates' food to binge, and then puke in the Barnes & Noble's restroom on the way to pawn their roommates' CDs to get more money to binge. They're doing what I came to the city to do: audition and dance. And for that, I am jealous.

By the time I receive my security pass, a small army of dancers has arrived, along with the annual camera crews who've come to capture the best, leggiest, but faceless, photo from the sea of long legs wrapped around the entire city block of Radio City Music Hall. Hundreds have come to audition, hoping to obtain one of the few coveted open slots.

I'm in the first pack of fifteen or so dancers who've been sardined into the elevator to travel up to the seventh floor where the magic of the Radio City rehearsals take place. On our walk down the long narrow hallways, through the maze to the rehearsal studio, it's impossible not to notice the beautiful pictures of former Rockettes that adorn Radio City's historic walls. Photographs of women dressed in classic Bob Mackie red-jeweled outfits with white-fur trim, standing in the perfect bevel, while others are linked arm-to-arm, eye-high kicking in green-velvet ensembles and silver t-straps, their smiles as sparkly as their diamond studs. Dating all the way back to 1933, the photographs represent the history of an American tradition and world-famous organization. I'm in awe of the glamour. I want to be one of these girls.

First things first. To be allowed to step foot into the Large Rehearsal Hall, the studio where the Rockettes rehearse, you have to be granted entry by the gatekeeper standing behind a card table piled high with sign-up sheet, pictures, and resumes.

"Picture and resume here, then stand in line to be measured," the woman says, waiting for me to toss my stapled picture and resume onto the pile of others. Like waiting outside a hot nightclub, we stand in line hoping to look good enough and have the digits to get past the bouncer; except that Radio City doesn't care about the pictures or numbers on the IDs. They care about the 8 x 10 black-and-white photos and the number of inches you stand in height. Per their nonnegotiable guidelines, you must be between 5'6" and 5'10" tall. You could be the female equivalent to Baryshnikov; but if you don't measure up, you ain't gettin' in.

When it's my turn, I stand barefoot, as tall as I can, my chin held high, hoping it will provide me with another inch. I know I'm tall enough, but I'd like to be on the taller side of the height requirement.

"It looks like you're 5'7" tall," Miss Monitor says. I'll take it.

I grab a spot in the center of the room in front of one of the mirrored walls, and take off my warm-ups. I'm wearing a turquoise leotard, tan tights, and tan t-strap heels. It's the standard garb, although some are dumb enough to wear black-belled jazz pants or little hot shorts over their tan tights that interrupt and shorten every long line the judges are looking for. They want to see legs, people!

I stretch and I wait. Many more packs of fifteen have sequestered themselves to the rehearsal hall. Around the room, huddles of cliques chat it up, as if they don't have a care in the world. As they laugh and carry on, however, I see them measuring up the competition from the corner of their eyes as their neighbor stretches or practices pirouettes. I, of course, do this too.

"Numbers one through fifty come into the Large Rehearsal Hall," the gatekeeper shouts. That's my cue.

I walk into the studio and drop my dance bag in a corner, making sure my number "3" is securely safety-pinned across the center of my leotard before racing to get the best audition spot—precisely front and center of the judges' table. I smile confidently, looking into each pair of eyes of the four I need to impress: Mark, the director, Lynn, the Rockette choreographer, and the two assistants.

After the requisite "Welcome and Good Luck" speech that happens at all auditions, we begin to learn choreography. I should probably mention that I do have a slight advantage. I've been a Rockette before. No, not in New York, but in the CONY shows, Christmas Outside of New York. This confuses people, who think that there's one Radio City clan that tours from city to city. Not true. Depending on the year, there are five to six casts of Radio City Rockettes deposited in each city. The line consists of eighteen dancers, plus two swings, in case someone is sick or hurt.

For the last two seasons, I performed in Branson, Missouri. At first I thought, Branson? With entertainment limited to the likes of *The Osmonds* or *The Andy Williams Show*, and shopping amidst the droves of seniors in search of homemade fudge and antique dolls, I thought it would be a drag. With exception to the constant bingeing I did before, between, and after shows, it actually ended up being a sweet gig. We lived in timeshare condos, were provided cars, were treated like celebrities, and regularly stopped by the locals to sign autographs at the in-town Wal-Mart. Branson is only a couple of hours from where I grew up in Kansas City, so it was nice to have my family and friends see me perform.

The New York show holds much more clout, simply because of its locale and the history of Radio City Music Hall. Then, there is the issue of the Rockette Roster. The Rockette Roster is a list, unique to the New York show, which has the status of tenure in academia, but causes the cattiness of a high school clique. The roster has been around forever, providing those in this privileged, chosen group job security and first dibs on any and every publicity event during the holiday season, such as kicking with Katie Couric on *The Today Show* or performing in the Macy's Thanksgiving Day Parade.

Although several of the routines are the same in both the New York and CONY shows, all of the choreography they're throwing at us this morning is new to me. It's only fair, really, as there are many other CONY dancers auditioning. I've always been a quick study, so I'm not worried. After learning a tap and jazz combination, and a kick line, they call us to audition.

"Okay, we're going to begin. We'll call you out in groups of four. When you hear your name, stand over here," the assistant choreographer says, pointing to the black *X*s taped onto the hardwood floor.

"Heather Beeman, Carlie Smith, Greta Gleissner, and Rosanne Connely," she announces. I scurry out to the floor and find my marker. Luckily, I'm in the middle.

"Okay, the piano will play two bars, then you'll begin," the director says.

Sixteen bars later, my audition is finished. It has gone well. I hit every beat, turn, and kick, all with the precision and perfection that the job demands.

After being sent to the Small Rehearsal Hall to wait for the remaining four or five groups of fifty to audition, finally it's time for the results.

"If we call your number, please come back for callbacks. If not, thank you for coming and please try again next year," says Lynn, the Rockette choreographer.

Holding a stack of pictures and resumes, she starts calling numbers, from highest to lowest.

"48, 43, 42, 36 . . . 16, 10, 4, 3, 1." Yes! She called my number! "Congratulations for making it through this round of auditions," she continues. "We'll see you in two weeks for callbacks."

I am a step closer to fulfilling my dream.

TWO WEEKS PASS, and I, along with forty-nine other women, return to the Large Rehearsal Hall, ready to conquer our final audition. This time, Eileen Collins, the head honcho of Radio City Productions is here to observe all of the remaining competitors, the crème de la crème, so to speak. She has us perform the same combinations we learned at the first audition, and I fly through the tap and the jazz competition without a problem. They make another cut.

Now down to twenty-five women—all of us still unclear as to how many they're looking for—we perform a final kick line in groups of five. After four groups, it's my turn to kick. This is it, the make-or-break final performance of the afternoon.

I stand in a bevel waiting for the piano to play, with my chin held high, a bright smile, and arms linked with the women on either side of me. I glide through the combination. Everything's going perfect until I feel a heel dig into my shin from the leg of the flustered girl next to me. *YOOUUU . . . BITCH!!!!* I smile through my fury, remaining unaffected on the surface, all the while thinking about how I'm going to kick, not her leg, but her ass if I lose this job because she fucked up!

The panel of four sends us back to the Small Rehearsal Hall while they deliberate.

I feel a tap on my shoulder. "Sorry about that." It's the girl who kicked me.

"Oh, that's okay, it happens," I reply. My smile is warm, but my insides are still hot with rage at her mishap. These things only "happen" if you're a complete idiot.

"Okay, everyone, please come back into the studio," one of the assistants directs.

Oh my God, it's time.

"We're going to put you into two groups. If I call your name, go back to the Small Rehearsal Hall."

My name isn't called. Several dancers from the CONY shows are asked to go into the other room. I have no idea what this means for me. The only girl I know in my room is Becky, a Rockette from the Branson show. Seeing all of those girls who are so much prettier than me escorted out, I'm sure I'm in the group about to be snipped of the chance to perform at Radio City. Lynn takes the girls whose names were called into the other room. The rest of us wait in the

Large Rehearsal Hall in silence. A few minutes later, Lynn comes back into the room.

"First, I'd like to say thank you to all of you for coming to the audition today," Eileen Collins begins. Great. Here it comes, we're about to be cut.

She continues. "I'd also like to say that we look forward to you performing in the *Radio City Christmas Spectacular* for the upcoming holiday season. You are our new Radio City Rockettes. Congratulations."

Yes! I made it!! Out of hundreds who auditioned, I, the girl who feels too ugly to even look at her face in the mirror, have been one of the ten chosen to be a New York Radio City Rockette. Wow. Pure satisfaction. I walk out of the Music Hall elated. Finally, I can dance in the city I love.

Now, I just have to get my eating under control.

To kick off my new life of success and health, I pop into the deli down the block for a salad. The salad bar is exquisite, as it should be for $6.99 a pound. Don't these produce price gougers know how heavy salad and its accoutrements are? A salad will be the perfect choice. Well, that's not entirely true. Salad creates, for me, this kind of empty full feeling, leaving me unsatisfied and bloated, which 99 percent of the time triggers me to throw up. *Not today. It's my new life. I can handle it.*

To ensure salad digestion, I decide on the way into the deli what my salad will consist of: Romaine, turkey, red peppers, and fat-free balsamic vinaigrette. It's nothing exciting, but clearly, I can't handle exciting food. I pick-up the silver salad tong, claw into the tin of Romaine lettuce, and grab a hefty portion. I toss a few squares of oven-roasted turkey into the mix. I prefer smoked, but bland oven-roasted will have to do. I can't help but notice the Gorgonzola crumbles and hunks of avocado staring at me as I bypass them to grab my red peppers. *Maybe I can have a little Gorgonzola.* No, I already decided. I snatch a few red peppers with a small tong and throw them onto my bed of Romaine. My eyes slide back over to the avocados. *Avocado, now that's a good fat. I can have some of that. The official food pyramid says so. Adults every day are supposed to eat a small amount of good fats like avocados, almonds, flaxseeds, and all of those other Omega-packed foods.* I know better. It may be a good fat, but avocados aren't a part of my "good," meaning allowed, foods. I'm stumped. I don't know what to do. If I eat the avocado, it might feel foreign to my stomach, which will trigger me to binge and purge. If I don't eat the avocado, I might wind up feeling completely unsatisfied by the lack of substance in my salad, which will cause me to purge anyway. I'd better eat the avocado.

These are the games I play with myself. I'm in a constant state of contemplation. Do I or don't I? What will happen if I do? Or don't? It's always about how I might feel in the future. Whatever I decide, even with the best of intentions, I seem to pick the wrong choice most of the time. My life centers on trying to find the most emotionally fulfilling foods to eat that won't make me feel too full or too fat, the goal being to prevent any level of physical discomfort, which is the ultimate trigger of a bulimic episode. Emotionally fulfilling foods, for me, are anything with gobs of cheese, sugar, chocolate, and/or creaminess. From where I sit, I'm screwed because I can never eat these foods without feeling full or fat, along with the fact that any food, or drink for that matter, can make me feel full enough or fat enough to give me a credible excuse to puke.

I throw a glob of scrumptious avocado into my container, staining the purity of my salad. At this point, I'm still telling myself that adding this bit of glistening green delight to my salad is okay; but in the pit of my being, where my only shreds of honesty exist, I know this move has given me the green light to purge. I only need one excuse, and now I have one. *Hmm . . . maybe I should grab a little Gorgonzola.* I'll eat a healthier salad next time. I know I'm going to purge. I'll have to start anew tomorrow.

Every time I build a salad, I tell myself to just get the balsamic vinaigrette. In my entire life, I've never gotten the balsamic vinaigrette. Vinaigrette is so boring and tasteless, compared to its creamy counterparts like ranch and blue cheese. My decision process is like buying stocks: I weigh all of my options, looking at different portfolios, and know that if I take too many aggressive risks, I'll crash and burn. I've already screwed up, so what the hell. I shower my salad with ranch dressing. In less than a minute, my salad has gone from a potpourri of purity to an adulterated pile of saturated fat.

I sit down at one of the deli tables to eat. I bulldoze through my salad. I can't tolerate the physical fullness even after a few bites. I have to throw up. But I can't because there isn't a bathroom for me to use. Well, there is, but it's reserved for employees. Compared to other cities that I've binged and purged in, the bleak New York bathroom situation requires an extra level of strategizing.

I hop on the subway, sitting amongst ostensibly emotionless people with blank stares, paying no attention to the blind accordion player or the legless veteran hand-walking his way along the skanky subway floor begging for money. I get off at Columbus Circle and head toward Broadway Dance Center where I'm taking class in about an hour. More importantly, there's a restroom. I take the elevator up to the fifth floor. Dancers all around, behind the check-in counter or stretching on the floor, greet me. They know me. They should, I've taken class daily for the last two years. Not to mention, I'm one of Michele's class assistants. Michele is one of the most renowned teachers in the country.

I dart to the restroom. It has two stalls. One is occupied, so I go into the unoccupied stall and stand with my feet facing forward—as if I'm actually going to go to the bathroom—and wait for the dancer next to me to finish. Waiting is the worst part. As soon as I hear the flush of her toilet, I turn around as fast as I can and lean over to perform a controlled quiet purge while her toilet is still sucking and swallowing. A move that requires impeccable timing. By the splatters around the toilet, I know I'm not the only bulimic who has been here today. I keep an ear out for the swinging of the bathroom door, for the entrance of newcomers, my signal to scoot my feet back around as fast as I can to the front and repeat the same waiting game. I do three sets of this dance before I feel empty enough to stop.

I come out of the bathroom, go to the sink to wash my hands, and look at my face, into my eyes. I don't show any signs of someone who just threw up. *You did it again. You told yourself you wouldn't and you did. You'll have to start fresh tomorrow.* The problem is that tomorrow never comes. *You just have to be stronger. Forget about it for now. You just made the New York Radio City Rockettes for God's sake! Be happy for yourself!* Clearly, the voices in my head could stand to lighten up; but the perennial question is "How?"

I go to the snack bar area and buy a Balance Bar and Diet Coke. I hear my name called from across the room.

"Hey, Greta, come here for a sec," Shirley, the office manager says. I walk over to her.

"A guy from ABC called and they need a couple of dancers for *All My Children*. I thought you and Mara could do it. Are you interested?"

"Are you kidding? That's my favorite soap opera! Of course I'll do it!"

"Here are the details. Call the casting director. He wants to meet with you guys to discuss the shoot."

Two jobs in one day! And I'm going to be on television! This is how I envisioned my life as a dancer. Besides the earlier salad mishap, my day couldn't be any better. A subtle anxiety starts kicking in. *The job is in one month. That's perfect. If I cut five hundred calories from my diet, and I burn five hundred calories exercising a day, I can lose eight pounds by the time of the shoot. I can do that.* These racing thoughts are what I tell myself to justify a pervasive notion: I have to look skinny, always, at all costs.

Class starts at 6:15 PM. I always arrive at least fifteen minutes early so that when the class before Michele's lets out, I can dash across the floor to my spot, in the front right corner of the studio. During my first year in the CONY shows, my friend Anne told me that when I moved to the city I should take classes with Michele, that I was her type of dancer. She was right. From the moment I stepped foot into her class, I loved it, and I quickly became one of her assistants. I can't help but blurt out my news about becoming a Rockette. Everyone congratulates me, making me feel like the class VIP for a moment.

After class, Michele and a group of us go out for sushi. During dinner, Michele mentions something about a teaching gig in Italy she's doing in August. Everyone else at the table knows what she's referring to, as they have all been asked to go. Immediately, I feel rejected. Why doesn't she think to ask me? *Hello, Dummy. She didn't ask you because you're an ugly, fat loser.* Maybe if I was prettier, if I was thinner. After hinting that I want to go, Michele invites me. I feel embarrassed for weaseling my way in, but I know that to lament over hearing for the next three months about an Italy trip I wouldn't be going on would make me feel much worse.

This is the story of my life. I'm good, but not good *enough*. I am talented, but I don't have *enough* of a look. I am a technical dancer with not *enough* style. I've had moments of brilliance, but not *enough*. I can perform the steps, but I don't provide *enough* emotion. My shackles of self-loathing and insecurity don't allow me to be free *enough*.

I'm like a chocolate soufflé that never fully rises to the occasion. It tastes good, the ingredients are all there, but the look is off just enough that it can't be served as the final course at a dinner party.

I excuse myself to go to the restroom to throw up. Throwing up is definitely something I do enough.

AFTER DINNER, I hop on the train downtown and get off at Fourteenth Street. I live in prime Greenwich Village just a block from the subway. My street is filled with glorious townhouses and quaint restaurants on the garden levels of brownstones.

Sandwiched between these eighteenth-century homes sits a big brown building, the Markle Residence. Otherwise known as the Salvation Army, the Markle Residence is a women's home filled mostly with performers and students who go to schools like Fashion Institute of Technology, The New School, and Marymount Manhattan College. In the summertime, young talented bun heads studying ballet at the Joffrey Ballet School stay for weeks, which is how I found out about it many years ago when I studied there. Besides women, a small percentage of the population is senior citizens. And if you're a man over sixty-five, then you can live in this women's residence.

I walk into the Markle trying to avoid the rude front desk attendants and head toward the elevators. The Markle mostly is run by employees from the West Indies. They attend the lobby, clean our rooms, and serve our food. They do their jobs with languid alacrity, with any resident request taken as a great imposition.

Included in our monthly rent are two meals a day. The setup is cafeteria style, with the employees doling out our miniscule portions. When I go through the line I always want less of this, more of that. *No. You can only have one serving of mashed potatoes.* The staff doesn't allow for substitutions, and given that my nickname since adolescence has been "Special Order," you can imagine the daily power struggles I go through.

One area I do have control over is the salad bar. I can eat as much salad as I want. I pile it as high as I can, drowning it in Russian and blue cheese dressing, before making my way to the communal tables. Each day I do the same routine: eat, purge in the dining room bathroom; eat, purge in the dining room bathroom, over and over. Eating disorders aren't prevalent in the West Indies, but the employees aren't dummies. They despise me because they know what I do with food. With every round trip I make from the salad bar to the bathroom and back to the salad bar, the rolling of their eyes shame me. *Yes*, I want to say, *I, too, am ashamed of myself.*

I take the elevator up to my room on the fifth floor. For the price of $580 a month, I share a quad, otherwise known as a small fucking room, with three women, Amy, Jennifer, and Annie. Amy is a fair-skinned brunette preppy whose Club Monaco wardrobe makes her look like she's ready to scoot off to the Hamptons at any moment. She stays at her boyfriend's apartment much of the time, is often snobby, and answers questions with condescension. Her voice changes to a high-pitched whine when she grows angry with me for eating her Luna Bars.

Jennifer is a student at Alvin Ailey. We get along great. We'll go out together often to show off our dance moves to members of the band as we dance onstage at Café Wha?. She's in class or at rehearsal at least five days a week, so she's hardly ever home.

I met my third roommate Annie years ago when I was on scholarship at Tremaine Dance Center in North Hollywood. Now we're both in the city living together in our quad, which is a duo about 70 percent of the time. My roommates are all aware of my eating disorder, but they mostly tiptoe around it.

I walk into my room, hoping my other three roommates are not home. Below my friendly exterior, I'm an introvert at heart. I'm not sure if it's a function of depression, or just an innate characteristic, but I require a lot of alone time. With juggling of dance classes and work, I can't wait to have some down time to do nothing. Unfortunately, I always ruin it by bingeing and purging, which tires me.

"Hi, Annie," I say. Thank God she is the only one home.

"Hey, what's up? How'd the audition go?" Annie has a rich brown tone to her skin, the type that doesn't seem to require sunscreen, and great wild frizzy hair. She has the type of ethnic look that Los Angeles dance jobs often require, and that I never had.

"Well, I made it! And, I also was asked to do a job for *All My Children*. It isn't for a couple of months and Radio City isn't until September, but at least I have some jobs lined up." I feel pretty proud of myself. For dancers, making the Rockettes isn't a big deal. It's just another gig. Plus, it isn't what dancers call *real* dancing. It's *precision* dance. Whatever you want to call it, the audition is competitive and the job pays really well. For that I feel proud.

"Oh my God, that's awesome."

"How was your day?" I ask, throwing my dance bag on my bed.

Within our dingy room are two sets of bunk beds. I'm afraid of heights, so I sleep on the bottom. Adorning the walls are a dresser and desk for each of us. Between the carpet, which hasn't been washed in God knows how long, and the used dark furniture, the room is one big blob of shit-color brown.

I often wonder if the furniture serves as a protective factor for rodent control. Rumor has it that the residence has failed past inspections because of problems with mice and roaches. My perfected defense of denial comes in handy when I hear people use the words mice droppings and food in the same sentence. Luckily, I don't digest much of the food.

"My day was alright. I got a job."

"Oh, yeah? What is it?" I ask. Annie has done odd jobs since she moved to the city, working in this restaurant or that nightclub. I actually don't know why she's in New York. From what she told me, she just needed a change. New York is hard enough to deal with when you have a purpose. Without one, I'm not sure what the point is. But, I guess she'll figure it out.

"I'm going to deliver pot."

"What? Really? How much do you get paid?" I had heard about these underground jobs, but had never known anyone who actually had one.

"$200 for eight hours, or $100 for four hours." Annie doesn't seem concerned that this is something completely illegal.

"That's cool. Does it make you nervous at all, ya know, carrying all that pot around?"

"No, they've been in business for a while and haven't gotten busted. The only way to become a customer is through referral, so it's pretty safe."

I haven't smoked pot since I lived in Los Angeles in the mid-nineties. I had a job back then delivering Chinese food. I loved the flexibility and that I was paid to drive around in my car listening to music. But I certainly didn't make $200 a shift.

SOON AFTER MY Radio City audition, a clusterfuck of insanity begins. For starters, I cannot find a restaurant job I like. I have several months before the Radio City season starts, so I have to find a job to financially tide me over. Between upselling margaritas at the Mexican restaurant, serving dim sum and Pan-Asian cuisine at the Chinese restaurant, serving chicken parmesan at the Italian Bistro, and refilling Guinness' at the Irish bar and grill, I have binged, purged, and served my way around the world—all in the borough of Manhattan. While I convince myself that each restaurant gig I acquire and quit is the restaurant that will allow me to work without eating and purging before, during, or after my shift, they all prove disastrous for my healthy eating goals.

My eating patterns at the Markle are growing progressively worse. Even the senior citizens know what I am up to once I enter the television room with a bag from Food Emporium or Duane Reade drugstore. I also can't pay my weekly rent on time, due to all of the money I spend on Hershey's Kisses, Hostess Ho Hos, and the like. I have to find a way that will allow me the flexibility to take class, go to auditions (as if I'll actually go), make money to pay my bills, and not binge and purge. The problem with the performing arts and living in NYC is that one of the only jobs that allow this is the restaurant business. It's the fastest way to make cash.

I still dance. Because I am one of the class assistants, Michele often allows me to take classes free of charge. Dance is the one place where I find peace. Well, in between trying to not be overshadowed by the next shining star that can walk into the studio at any moment. Everyone knows Michele, so you never know who is going to pop in and steal the attention.

While I love dance class, my feelings of insecurity steal much of the joy I would otherwise receive. My motivation during warm-up and progressions and turns across the floor stems from the hit of adrenaline and self-esteem that comes from the glance, smile, or comment said by the teacher leading the class. Of course, I harangue myself for being aware of this. All I want to do is stop worrying about what others think, and dance for myself. But if I receive no praise, forget it, it's an automatic excuse for me to binge and purge my sorrows away.

I do look forward to making my soap opera debut later in the summer and kicking at Radio City in the fall, but I have to find some other way to make money. If I can just find something for a couple of months to tide me over, then I won't have to ask my mom or dad for money. Annie seems to be having a good time at her job. She has flexibility and always has cash in her pocket. She hasn't gotten arrested for the sale or possession of marijuana yet. It seems to be a win-win situation.

One afternoon, after making $30 on a six-hour lunch shift, I am completely fed up. How is a person supposed to survive on $5 an hour in New York City? Desperate for a change, I reflect back to the conversation I had with Annie about her new job. Maybe pot delivery is something I could do.

"Are you sure you want to do this?" Annie asks me. "Chris is kind of funny about letting new people in."

"I need a change. I can't stand the thought of working in another restaurant."

The following day, Annie and I head to Chris's apartment. I'm in the Napa Valley of marijuana. There are bundles of the highest quality weed the city has to offer in a range of varietals, spread over a coffee table. A girl named Sarah is weighing out the pot and stuffing it into rectangular plastic capsules that are big enough to hold an ounce or two of marijuana. Instead of pinot noir and cabernet sauvignon, there are names like "AK-47," "White Widow," or "Purple Haze," each signifying a different varietal and high.

"Hi, I'm Sarah," the girl says. She is in her midtwenties and studious looking. Although this is apparently Chris's place, if that is his real name, she is the only one in the apartment.

"Hey," I say. I'm feeling nervous. What if I get caught or screw up somehow? What type of hoodlums will I be delivering to?

"Here you go, Annie," she says, handing her a walkie-talkie and twenty rectangular capsules. "Today you're Chicago." All of the phones are coded with names of major cities so no one can be traced. Sarah takes all of the daily orders and then calls the delivery people on their phones, based on their location in the city. The system indicates to me that they run a tight ship.

"Cool, thanks," Annie says, throwing the capsules into her backpack, which is accompanied by dryer sheets to deter the thick smell of marijuana.

"Do you want to smoke before you go?" Annie and Sarah take a few hits. I politely decline, as I don't take mood-altering drugs anymore. When I lived with Annie in Los Angeles, we used to smoke pot a lot. It was no big deal. I had no bad experiences with drugs at that point.

My problematic experiences with drugs started when I met Melissa while I was working at Swensen's Ice Cream store six years ago. Melissa was a twenty-year-old free spirit, who only shopped at thrift stores and strolled around in vintage adidas jogging suits and Converse kicks.

"What are you doing after work?" Melissa asked me one day.

"Not much. Just chillin'." If you consider bingeing and purging on the macadamia nut ice cream I am going to steal after the shift chillin'.

"Wanna hang?" She asked.

"Sure."

After our shift, we hopped in Old Blue, my 1986 Chrysler Le Baron, and headed to her house in the Hollywood Hills. I was excited. I had always wondered what those hill houses looked like on the inside. When we arrived, I was amazed by all of the masks hanging on the walls.

"My dad is a director of horror movies. He just directed a *Tales for the Crypt* show." This is no big deal for Melissa. After all, she was raised here. Many parents are directors or show-biz types. I'm impressed.

"So, do you party?" Melissa asked me.

"What type of party?"

"Crystal."

I had done crystal meth a couple of times in the past with one of my friends from dance. I never thought I would snort anything up my nose.

"Yes, I've done it a couple of times."

"Wanna do some now?"

"Sure."

From that day forward, we spent a lot of time hanging out, getting high. We became artists on meth, paying close attention and studying every line and angle of the cartoon characters we were trying to replicate. We called ourselves the Spun Spoofers, tweaked at every turn.

Eventually, I quit the Swensen's job to be a delivery driver at a popular California-style Chinese restaurant. Annie got a job there, too. We delivered to all the movie studios and nice houses in Laurel and Coldwater Canyons. I met many celebrities; though, every time I delivered to Jerry Seinfeld's office or had to wait in the lobby with one of the Wayans brothers, I felt embarrassed. I knew they were thinking: *You're an ugly, fat, pit-faced mess.*

Joe, my manager, liked crystal, too. Melissa, Joe, and I got high several times a week. A dance friend of mine, Lizzie, was into cocaine, so she partied with us also. It was one big powder and rock fest. The problem was when I became increasingly paranoid. I started believing the helicopters that regularly fly around Los Angeles at night were after me. I was constantly looking out of my apartment door peephole to see if a police officer was waiting to arrest me.

One night, after partying with Lizzie, I decided that I really needed to stop all the drugs, so I took the last of the crystal out of the mini-sized, clear, sealed baggie. As soon as I snorted it, I knew I had done too much. My body was buzzing, my heart racing. Instantly, paranoia set in, and I thought I was having a heart attack.

Lizzie took me to McDonald's for some orange juice. I hate orange juice, but somehow thought that it could solve the near-death experience I was having.

A few hours later, I had to work at the Chinese restaurant. It was the middle of summer and my car air conditioner was broken. Between the heat and my pseudoheart attack symptoms, there was no way I could deliver Chinese food. Annie, luckily, came in to help me. She took me into a grungy work closet, where I laid panic-stricken on the dirty floor, and convinced me in between her deliveries that I was not dying.

I lived to tell the story and vowed to never touch crystal again. Well, until two days later when I smoked it. And then I put it down for good.

Because of my experiences with crystal, I can no longer enjoy anything that's mood altering, which includes marijuana. Drugs make me feel too out of control. I am completely out of control with my food, but that doesn't make me paranoid. For some reason, the words "drug overdose" scare me much more than the words "esophageal hemorrhage," which I'm at risk for every time I throw up.

ANNIE TAKES ME on her marijuana deliveries for the day. To my surprise, the clientele is a mix of clean-cut wealthy types, models, and students. It seems like no big deal. This might be the perfect job for me. I would usually never do such a risky job, but my ultimate disdain for the restaurant business has left me desperate. I can't work an office job. Besides having no office skills, there is no way I can sit at a desk for eight hours a day. I'd feel trapped. Clearly, pot delivery is my next best move. *Sure, Greta. Even you don't buy that one.*

My first day out, I go to the apartment and collect my tools. Instead of an apron, a wine key, and a server book, I'm handed a "Dallas" walkie-talkie and many capsules of designer pot, taped shut by their funky designer labels. I shove them into a red and white-striped Estee Lauder makeup bag.

The high-pitched beep on my walkie-talkie lets me know I have my first delivery in Thompkins Square Park, a known drug haven. Great. I have never gone to the Alphabet City neighborhood and have only heard scary stories about it. Everywhere I walk, whether on the subway or on the street, I'm sure I have "Pot Deliverer" written across my forehead. I avoid police officers that scout the vicinity of the East Village. When I pass them, I smile and look them directly in the eyes to let them know that I'm just a normal girl, not a criminal.

As I make my way to Thompkins Square, I see two cops standing on opposite corners. As I walk closer, I notice their guns are drawn. My first thought is that they are waiting for me. Scenarios of imprisonment and "Drug Dealing Rockette" newspaper headlines zip through my mind. I begin to panic. One officer looks at me, his hand motioning for me to go away. I turn around and run the opposite direction, my heart racing, in fear of being caught in the crossfire.

I arrive at the client's apartment, covered in sweat, nervous to see who is going to answer the door for my first delivery. I peek into his apartment, which is a loft filled with modern décor.

"Hey," the man at the door says. By his beautiful appearance and perfect body he obviously is a model.

"Here you go," I say, handing him his two capsules.

"Thanks," he says. He's happy to see me, but not too into small talk. I imagine he's thinking, *I know I'm hot . . . but you . . . look at you and your big nose. You have no cheekbones on that pitted face of yours. Just give me the weed and go, fat ass.* There is only one purpose for my presence in his glam world. He opens it up and smells it. He's pleased. He hands me four $50 bills, and I'm on my way.

I did it. I made my first delivery. Sarah hasn't beeped me for my next delivery, so I head to Au Bon Pain by NYU. I indulge a small twenty-minute binge before Sarah beeps me for my next delivery. She directs me to head uptown to east Fifty-Third Street. I quickly purge in the bathroom before heading out. Looking in the mirror at myself in this dingy customer bathroom, I'm disgusted. I'm not a drug dealer. I'm a dancer. *How did my life come to this?*

After that first delivery, I know that this is not the job to cure my eating woes. Restaurant business or not, my eating disorder finds a way to slither its slimy self into my life and bite me with poisonous venom. The main problem isn't the bingeing. I actually don't love to stuff my face. *Well, maybe I do.* The problem is that nothing gives me as much pleasure and instantly reduces as much pain as purging does.

The final straw on my delivery business comes on a rainy April day. The city has been experiencing torrential downpours for a couple of days. I am hoping the rain will stop before I have to work, but, of course, it doesn't. Dread sets in. I hate getting wet. Beeeeep! Sarah's calling me. *Don't answer it. I have to. I hate my life.* Fifty-Eighth and First Avenue. I hate traveling to that area.

As I make the trek to First Avenue, a gust of wind pushes me backward. Remorse sets in as I think about all of the auditions I didn't go to when I felt fat and insecure and chose to binge instead. *You could've had a job instead of doing this shit. What's wrong with you? You dumb piece of shit.* A gale force overtakes my umbrella, and I duel the wind. The umbrella turns inside out. With no protection against the rain, I lose the battle. My entire body is soaked. I'm miserable.

Suddenly, a flash of a pizza slice enters my brain. Relief begins to comfort me; my lips form a half smile. Bingeing and purging on pizza is my ticket out. That's that—my days as a pot deliverer are finished. I ignore Sarah's beeps for the rest of the day, just like I'd ignored past restaurant managers' when I'd pulled my final no-show. I'll give my pot stash to Annie to return. I'm going to enjoy my pizza.

SCENE 2

A Spectacular Life

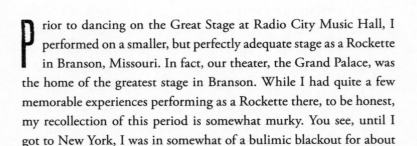

Prior to dancing on the Great Stage at Radio City Music Hall, I performed on a smaller, but perfectly adequate stage as a Rockette in Branson, Missouri. In fact, our theater, the Grand Palace, was the home of the greatest stage in Branson. While I had quite a few memorable experiences performing as a Rockette there, to be honest, my recollection of this period is somewhat murky. You see, until I got to New York, I was in somewhat of a bulimic blackout for about a decade.

When looking back at photo albums, reminiscing about my two years in Branson, my mother will see a picture of me and will begin to rattle off a string of bright memories.

"Oh, Greta, remember when we went shopping and we sang Christmas carols and toured the Candy Cane house?" she'd ask.

Huh? Sadly, I only have a vague idea of what she's talking about. It's almost as if I wasn't even there. My mind was obsessed with things like how my stomach was sitting on my jeans, the mental torture that came when offered a sample of fudge, and how I was going to keep food down or find a bathroom to get rid of it without my parents knowing.

What I remember are bits and pieces. It's much like a blackout alcoholic who drives home drunk, but doesn't remember how he got there. Oh, he might remember a glimmer of the experience, like sitting in his car and wondering if he'd make it home alive, or almost slamming into the car in front of him on the off-ramp of the interstate, but the rest of the experience will be cloudy, at best. I wasn't in a literal blackout, like in alcoholism. It was mental obsession that led me to miss the details and experiences of my daily life, such as keeping up with what I ate, what I was going to eat, if I needed to purge, where I could purge, how my stomach felt, how fat I felt, how full I felt, if I exercised enough, etc. What a waste.

IN OCTOBER, ON my twenty-fifth birthday, rehearsals for the *Christmas Spectacular* begin. A couple of days before, my stepfather drove me to Springfield, Missouri, to my new home, which is a room at the Extended Stay Hotel. I don't know what to expect when I walk into the Grand Palace rehearsal hall that first day. I am excited. I made the role of Rockette, which is a professional milestone; and also I am envisioning the close friendships I will make as the cast of entertainers becomes like extended family.

Because auditions are over, I naively believe we are all on equal, three-inch high-heeled footing. I quickly realize, however, that while the auditions are in the distant past, a thick, concentration of competitive air pollutes the hall. I and at least a half a dozen others are now the "new girls." Many of the dancers have been Rockettes for years. I am completely green, knowing none of the pieces or the ins and outs of performing as a Rockette. I'm also replacing a dancer, so I imagine they are comparing me to her.

Some of the women are extremely open and nice, while others look the other way when I smile at them. Some just stare with judging eyes. *Ignore it, Greta. Don't be intimidated.* I know that I wouldn't have been chosen if I wasn't good enough. My eyes scan the other women. I am different. Most of the girls have very long hair and perfect complexions, while I have short, white blond hair and cheeks full of little icepick indentations from years of acne. I know that everyone has something they don't like about themselves. I would have much preferred to have freckles. Or rosacea. A familiar sinking feeling invades my body. *Once again, Greta. You suck. You're so ugly. You probably just barely made it. You're the weak link.* One thing I know though, I am skinny. I'm fifteen pounds lighter than when I auditioned seven months ago.

Before I received the telephone call inviting me to be a CONY Radio City Rockette, I had been living with my Grandma Sally, who was dying from lung disease. I moved in with her after completing a six-month stint dancing on a cruise line. Though I sailed through Europe, the Panama Canal, went to Jerusalem, and saw the pyramids in Egypt, I spent most of my time bingeing and purging. I don't know if you've ever been on a cruise ship, but the food scene is a bulimic's nirvana or Dante's seventh circle of hell, depending on the day.

My bulimia had taken a serious turn sometime between Europe and the transatlantic crossing en route to the Bahamas. I had thrown up so much that I no longer had to force myself. By the time I arrived back home, I was purging five to ten times a day. Ice cream. Purge. Pasta. Purge. Diet Coke. Purge. Salad. Purge. Water. Purge. I couldn't keep a lot down.

Due to my constant bingeing and purging, I had pretty much eaten my way out of being welcome at my mother or my father's house. No one ever said I was unwelcome. It was a timing issue, really. Someone needed to help take care of Grandma Sally and I needed a place to stay. I was closer to Grandma Sally than most people in the family, so I was the natural choice. I didn't mind. I loved Grandma Sally.

Nothing changed about my bingeing and purging; what changed at Grandma Sally's was that in addition to taking dance classes daily, I also began a strict exercise regimen. I ran on the treadmill six miles a day and, within a couple of months, lost about twenty-five pounds.

When I went to dance class or work, my grandmother had additional help from her wonderful neighbor, Rosemary. One day, Rosemary was looking for something in the closet of the bedroom I was staying in and found my stash of vomit-filled plastic cups. Typically, I'd gather the cups into a large black plastic bag, haul them out to my car late at night and throw them in the trunk, like a dead body about to be tossed into a swampy river by mobsters. I had grown lazy.

When I came back from dance that night, there was a note attached to one of the cups: "Greta, you are out of control. Get control of yourself."

What the fuck? That bitch! Who is she to tell me anything?! She's just the neighbor. Rosemary, like a good neighbor, told my family, and soon after, I was off to the eighth-floor eating disorder ward at Baptist Memorial Hospital, in Kansas City, Missouri.

I gained ten pounds by the time I leave the hospital. When I'm discharged, I have a packet of CONY Rockette information regarding contractual obligations, rehearsals, performances, etc., waiting for me. I also received a two-page worksheet requesting all types of measurements. The only ones that matter to me are my height (5'7"), weight (123 lbs.), waist (25"), and hips (33"). I secretly wish I can be my prehospital weight, and hope that rehearsals help me shed those pounds.

Now in rehearsals, as these girls dart their derisive glances in my direction, I wonder if I look like someone recently released from an eating disorder unit. Can they tell that only weeks ago I was not allowed to go to the bathroom after meals without the accompaniment of a psychiatric nurse? Do they know that after I'd go to sleep each night, there'd be a flashlight shining on my face every thirty minutes to make sure I was okay? Will my thin frame tell them that I had to leave my hospital room door open to ensure that I wasn't compulsively exercising; that my meals were monitored to make sure I wasn't hiding my green beans in my napkin; or that I'd had a full-blown mental breakdown when being forced to drink an Ensure? I certainly hope not. After all, I'm here to forget about my past and start a new, healthier life. *Ha, ha, ha. Good one, Greta.*

Rehearsals are practically an extension of auditions. Every day, there's a team of people watching our every move. Linda Haberman, our director, is a drill sergeant. She was one of Bob Fosse's dancers and assistants. She walks in the rehearsal studio with her standard uniform, black leggings, a baggy sweater of some sort, and her Dansko clogs. The clogs are her signature piece. She owns many different styles and colors. She has short reddish brown hair and a hard face, and it's rumored that she is a lesbian. Repeatedly, she screams at us, "No!! Do it again!!!" Sometimes she mocks our movement when she demonstrates how we perform the choreography versus how she expects it to look. She is completely scary, but I absolutely love her. She is why we are great.

Like every other authority figure that has entered my world, I want to please Linda. She's hard to please, especially when I'm not exactly the most graceful with props. In the ragdoll routine, there are these oversized alphabet boxes that we twirl with one hand, while tap dancing at the same time. We also tap dance on top of the boxes, and then by the end of the routine, we end up in a line that spells out the words, "Merry Christmas."

There are specific techniques to how much you have to tilt the box and where the corner of the box needs to rest in the palm of your hand, so that it twirls the right way for the right amount of time and doesn't fall on the stage with a loud thud. Each side of the box has a letter on it, to ensure that the boxes don't spell out gibberish like, "Merxr Cjrimstsa," each dancer has a specific direction in which they must place the box on the ground. In rehearsal, Linda is irritated with me because I can't twirl my box. Until I develop the twirl technique, that damn box brings me to tears. Linda hisses at me and anyone else who flubs up, and then we have to do the number again. She's tough, but sometimes a smile peaks through her mask of irritation, signaling that she likes me.

How you look and perform on the Rockette line determines if you get extra work doing publicity events. There are meet-and-greets with the audience, performances on television morning shows, interviews, sports events, and photo shoots. Doing anything outside of our contractual twelve-shows-per-week agreement means extra money.

Through media training, I learn that public speaking is definitely not my forte, so that's out. I am able to do a few things here and there, like perform at a football game and be in the photo spread of a local Branson magazine. *Big whoop. I may have the body, but the bottom line is that I'm just not as pretty or as dazzling as some of the other girls.*

Of course, during my first year as a Rockette, I get sandwiched between the two most pretentious and immature girls on the line, Terri and Kelsy. During rehearsal, Terri would roll her eyes at me and say, "Greta, can you stop pushing my back when we kick?" From an audience's perspective, when we do a kick line, it appears that each dancer is holding onto the girl's backs next to them, to help support our line. In actuality, we barely touch the girls next to us, if at all. The reason being is that if we are using the dancers on either side of us for support, then the line will sway back and forth.

Kelsy, on the other hand, keeps her mouth shut. Instead, when I smile in her direction, her eyes speak harshly to me: *Don't smile at me. I don't like you. Get over yourself.* I don't want to be friends with such a fucking snob anyhow.

Once the show begins, the real test of endurance kicks in. While we are contracted for twelve shows a week, supposedly performing an average of two shows per day with one day off, we are actually performing three and sometimes four shows a day at the height of the season, due to the growing popularity of the show between Thanksgiving and Christmas. To mentally prepare, after I perform the first two shows, I go into the third acting as if I've just arrived to work. I also try to mentally block the two bulimic episodes that inevitably occur by the time I've performed two shows. If I would have actually taken the time to think about the number of shows I'd performed and the amount I'd purged by midafternoon, I'd probably pass out.

Performers on Broadway often complain about performing eight shows a week—what a cakewalk! During the show, however, there are many excruciating moments when I feel sure I'll never make it through without dying from exhaustion. Of course, I suffer in silence. I don't want to be talked about like Justine is.

Justine is this annoying little pill from Kentucky, whose claim to fame is that her uncle is a famous politician. Oh, and how could I forget, she's a beauty queen. While miss prim and proper carries herself gracefully off stage, whenever she is tired during the show she starts spewing profanities as well as saliva onto her Rockette Red lipstick (yes, it's really a color) through her pageant-perfect smile. A new diagnostic label could be created for her in the *Diagnostic and Statistical Manual of Mental Disorders*: Tourette's syndrome during periodic episodes of eye-high kicking.

In Justine's defense, Christmas in New York, the closing piece of the first act, is a beast. Ninety-nine kicks are required in that number, including the kicks in the Sit-Down Drill. The Sit-Down Drill is a kick series that the line performs while sitting on a bench. Occurring about halfway through the twelve-minute number, it would appear to the audience like a nice little breather. After all, we sit down to do our kicks, right? Wrong. It's a total ab- and hip-flexor workout. It should be proposed for a class at Equinox Fitness Club.

Once we stand up from the Sit-Down Drill, we move our way into our final kick line. It's the hardest series of the show, simply because there are so many damn kicks. As we do our final eight or ten kicks, I hear a voice near the end of the line. Obviously, I can't turn my head to look. Then I hear the familiar strain—Shit, fuck, I can't make it through! Fuck! I can't do it. Shit! Holy Shit! Fuck! I know just who it is. *There she goes.* Once again, Justine is cursing her way through the routine. Our smiles as we exit the stage leave the audience with an impression that we are just as sweet as the sugary scent of cinnamon pecans that float through the theatre. In reality, the Rockettes are scoffing at Justine behind her back. *What the fuck's wrong with her? We have to say something!* After huddling up and deciding to confront her, they blast her with a "You need to get a handle on yourself" speech. I wasn't about to be a Justine.

Little side events, like Justine's behavior, happen throughout each show without the audience ever knowing. During our numbers, the dancers and singers, particularly the gay boys backstage, wait in the wings and make obscene gestures in an effort to make us laugh when we turn toward them. Or the young ten-year-old boy in the show, who wished he could be a Rockette, would perform the choreography along with us, kicking in the wings. Whether observing these backstage antics from afar or participating in them myself, I did feel more connected at such times, more part of a family, even if only for a fleeting moment.

In the finale, The Living Nativity, we begin by walking behind the scrim, appearing in the shadows like peasants walking toward the promised land. While we walk, we have to be careful that we don't accidentally step into a smear of camel droppings. I try to walk across the stage holding my breath, the way I used to as a kid whenever my parents drove us past a graveyard. After all, the aroma of camel shit is, well, just plain shitty. Once we successfully navigate the turd mines, we come into full view onstage and then turn our backs to the audience, to salute Mary, Joseph, and baby Jesus.

It's a very beautiful number, and a crowd pleaser, especially in the Bible Belt of Branson where people are serious about their God. To the cast, it means only one thing, we are finally finished with the two-hour-and-fifteen-minute show. This is the time when I usually start deliberating with myself privately as to whether I'm going to binge or eat healthily during my break. Given the fact that I usually end up bingeing, maybe I really should be praying to God during the nativity scene instead of merely acting the part.

On occasion, before the nativity scene begins, many of us will take a black eyeliner pencil and blacken out one or two of our teeth. When Mary and Joseph look at us, we flash a big bum smile at them with our now-rotting teeth, trying to make them laugh. We have to do little tricks like that, because without actual dance steps to perform dancers and singers become extremely bored. We have to entertain ourselves in some way. The performers who play Mary and Joseph are professionals and never break character, but we can see in their eyes that they want to.

MY FAMILY LOVES that I am performing in Branson because it's so close to their own homes. My entire family—parents, stepparents, aunts, uncles, grandmother, cousins—come to watch me perform. Certain family members have been a little obsessed with anything that resembles fame, so they are delighted that I'm part of a world-renowned and seemingly glitzy troupe.

The sparkle in my dad's eyes tells me he's proud of me. It isn't that I never thought he was proud of me growing up; but he never could let himself be a part of my childhood passion because of the tension he felt toward my mother. Now, though, I feel like a star in his eyes. His inquisitiveness about the "little people," camels, and awe about our quick costume changes tell me that I finally have captured his attention.

My mother, too, is ecstatic. I think she's always wanted to dance professionally, so it's fun for her to be a part of my world. My mother tells everyone—her colleagues at work, friends, stylist, tap instructor—that I'm a Rockette.

Performing as a Rockette brings out creativity in several members on my mom's side of the family. My Stepuncle Ken is a professional sculptor, artist, and photographer. My Stepdad Kent commissioned him to make a two-foot bronze Rockette statue for my mother and me. My Cousin Jacqlyn used my performance as a Rockette for her role-model writing assignment at school. My Grandma Patty, a superb painter (who only began painting in her seventies!) painted a Rockette portrait from a picture of me posing in one of my costumes. No one would've thought that the Dixie Bell Dancer from years past would've blossomed into such a talented professional. In this way, I am perfect to my family.

If my eating disorder was not present, I would be on cloud nine. Beneath the symptoms of bulimia is my core dysfunction: I don't believe I deserve any of the attention. I mean, how could I deserve anything given the awful things I do with food, and that my face is so ugly that it needs to be covered with makeup? I want to live the life of happiness I portray through my smile onstage, but my lack of self-worth and deep-seated sense of inadequacy never allow me to fully enjoy any of it.

Every day when the choreographers glance at me, I'm certain that they know they have made a big mistake. I'm sure that all of the girls on the line are wondering how I nabbed this job. I constantly focus on every negative quality I have.

AFTER MY FIRST season ends, I'm not sure if I want to return to the Radio City Rockette clan. Yes, I made friends, but it is all so political and competitive. I like performing, the money, and the perks that come with it, but overall I didn't have that great of a time. If I'm not invited back, I decide that I won't reaudition to be a Rockette again.

Instead, I audition for Tokyo Disney, and land the job! This means that I'll be spending ten months in Tokyo making quite a bit of money. As Tokyo grows closer, however, I worry about being in another country with an eating disorder. There's so much more to think about than just the normal adjustments, like converting dollars to yen. *What if my eating is out of control? Will I be able to binge? What will I binge on? Japanese snack cakes? Will I like them? What if I can't eat my brands of healthy food? What if I have a heart attack and die alone in Japan?*

These are concerns you think about as a professional bulimic dancer.

Weeks before I'm supposed to fly out, Japan has a massive earthquake. Having survived at the epicenter of a California earthquake years prior, I'm terrified. Between my eating and the quake, I decide there is no way I can go. I call the producers at Disney and use the eating disorder as a crutch to renege my contract.

Ironically, the following day, I receive a call from Radio City Productions asking me if I'd like to return to Branson to perform as a Rockette. Wow, I don't have to reaudition. I can't believe they like me enough to ask to back! Yes, of course, I will go. A couple of months later, I'm heading back to Branson.

From the moment my second season as a Rockette begins, I know that I'm going to have a better experience. Not being the new girl makes all the difference. Maybe I'll even speak well enough in the media training to do an interview. *Let's not push it, Greta.*

Like the first year, I arrive a couple of days early to the Extended Stay Hotel. Anytime I start a new job, a new school year, a new anything, I always believe it will be the elixir to cure my eating. *This time, I'm going to eat perfectly. I'm not going to binge and purge. I won't make the same mistakes.* Empty promises I seem never able to fulfill. Of course, on the very first night staying at the hotel, I think to myself, *I'll just binge and purge this once, and then never again for the rest of the season.*

I start eating, do a quick purge, and then decide to go buy ice cream. My stomach is still full, as I have not thrown up all the food I've eaten, but I know I'll only be gone a few minutes. As I begin to back my car out from its parking space, I see a girl walking up to me. I haven't met her, but I can tell by her dancer frame that she's part of the show. I really don't have time to talk to some random dancer, but I don't want to be rude. I roll down my window.

"Hey, I'm Autumn. I saw you walking out and wanted to introduce myself. Are you a Rockette or a dancer?"

"I'm Greta," I smile back. "I'm a Rockette. You?"

"I'm a dancer, one of the ballerinas," she says. "Is this your first year doing the show?"

Autumn looks like a ballerina. She has long thin arms with legs to match, and a beautiful long neck. My ballet mistress would've said she had the perfect facility. Her naturally blond hair falls gracefully onto her shoulders.

At this point, all I can think of is the binge food digesting and turning into fat in my stomach. I just want to drive to the ice cream shop and come home to purge. I don't know how I am going to get rid of this girl.

"This is my first year," she says. "I actually just came back from taking a break with dance. I'm going to die in rehearsals. I'm so out of shape! So, what are you doing now?"

Why does she want to know what I'm doing? Can't this girl leave me alone?

"Oh, I'm just going for an ice cream."

Autumn's piercing green cat eyes lock onto mine, and it's hard not to stare back into them. I turn away, though, hoping she will cue to my subtle hint that the buzzer on our chat time was over about two minutes ago.

"Cool, can I come?"

What? Is she serious? Come with me? Why? How will I binge on ice cream? More importantly, how will I purge?!

My gut, quite literally, is telling me to do anything but let her in the car. For some reason, I don't listen to it.

"Yeah, sure," I responded hesitantly. *Damn, Greta. Why'd you do that?*

My stomach feels like a water balloon about to pop.

As we drive, I can't help but wonder why she wants to come with me. On the way, we make small talk about the usual topics dancers talk about: the coast you live on, if you like it, what gigs you've been doing, who you take classes from. The ice cream shop has a drive-thru, so we each order a couple scoops of mint chip ice cream on sugar cones, and then head back to the hotel.

I step out of the car and walk over to the passenger side to wait for Autumn. When she climbs out, I start to walk toward the hotel, scooping up dripping bits of ice cream with my tongue. I feel a tug on my arm pulling me backward.

The next thing I know, I'm pressed up against the Ford Taurus with Autumn's lips attacking mine. Our cold, mint chip-coated tongues are dancing with one another. *Oh. My. God. Autumn is a lesbian!* So many things swirl through my head: First, I had no idea she was gay. Second, I can't believe that she thinks I'm gay! And third, I like kissing her.

For years, I've been contemplating my sexuality. From a young age, I had a sneaky suspicion that I was gay. I always wanted to like guys, but in high school I was never really interested, and certainly not boy-crazy like my friends. I was confused when my best friends started having sex. What was wrong with them? I wanted to continue wearing the made-for-two heart-shaped "Best Friend" necklaces we'd exchanged and wore around our necks. I wanted to be their special "other half," not some dumb boyfriend.

There was no way, however, that I could be gay in my family. My parents were complete homophobes. They thought that being gay was a mental disorder. Didn't they know that the American Psychiatric Association banished homosexuality as a mental disorder in 1973, the year I was born? (Interestingly, I was born on "National Coming Out" day.) None of us would've ever thought that twenty-some years later I'd be knowledgeable about the gay rights movement, or that I'd know the gay pride colors, or what a pink triangle signifies, or the various labels that differentiate the type of lesbian a person is. For the record, I'm a "lipstick lesbian."

To my parents, gay people were strange and had something wrong with them. My dad used to say things like, "Greta, how can you dance with those faggots?" or "Greta, he's a little light in the loafers, isn't he?" We did have one gay person in my family—my Grandma Sally's favorite uncle. The only two things I knew about his lifestyle is that he listened to Liberace and that his snake of a lover stole all of the money that my grandmother was to inherit when he died.

A mother's intuition, even in denial, is often on point. When I was sixteen years old, I had just ordered my quarter-pounder with cheese from the McDonald's drive-thru when my mother asked me, "Greta, why don't you date boys like your cousin does? You're not gay, are you?" *Fuck no. I'll never be gay when you ask me like that.*

I was nineteen the first time I really took a look at my sexuality. I had moved to Los Angeles on a dance scholarship at Joe Tremaine, one of the most popular studios in the city. Coming from the suburbs of Kansas, I had never been exposed to many gay people. Here, the dance students were free with their sexuality.

During this time, I developed my first infatuation with a girl. Her name was Natasha, and she was amazing. She was three years younger than me, but emotionally more mature. The dancers I knew who grew up in the city seemed to be more advanced emotionally. Natasha was the best dancer in class. Her flexibility and the way she was able to contort her body made her an anomaly. At sixteen, she was also openly gay. She wasn't the stereotypical butch dyke that ignorant people think of when they lump all gay women into the lesbian category. Her long, naturally curly brown hair and thin body defied the stereotype. She was beautiful. Her best friend, Tammy, was a couple of years older than me. She also was gay.

These girls were not friendly. They made fun of other dancers, had inside jokes throughout class, and would scoff at you if you smiled their way. I wanted, needed, to find a way into their circle because they were the best. I needed to be a part of the best. I wanted to be a part of a special group, not just a clique of average dancers. I did it by earning their respect through my dancing. Eventually, I started hanging with them before and after classes, smoking cigarettes on the patio, or going for coffee. Natasha knew I liked her and she was a huge flirt. She let me know that she never made the first move. How was I supposed to make the first move?

That year, when my mother visited me, she wondered why all of my friends were gay. "Greta," my mom started. "Aren't they strange?" Strange was code for gay. "Yes," I said. My mom just looked at me, half confused, half suspecting. I didn't think she really wanted to know at that time that her daughter was gay, and I certainly wasn't ready to tell her.

A few years later, a distant relative on my father's side confessed that he'd been sleeping with his best friend, Anthony, for several years. At the dinner table, I'd hear all about his "mental disorder" and how he could've behaved differently if he chose differently. I was conflicted by my own feelings, and wondered if my family would think I had a mental disorder when I finally came out.

In my early twenties, I had a number of flings with women while I was under the influence of alcohol. Alcohol was the separation between the denial I lived sober and the reality I knew within me. There was my Jewish anorexic friend, whom I met in the hospital. After a brief fling with me, she fled to Israel and married a rabbi to escape her own mental disorders. On the cruise ship, my Canadian roommate and I had intoxicated flings, after which she'd escape back to her magician boyfriend. During the Christmas cruise, a male singer in my cast propositioned me. He wanted to watch me have sex with his girlfriend, Audrey, who was also a singer in the cast. Once we all sobered up, they went back to their heterosexual relationships and I went back to bingeing on tiramisu.

After that first kiss in the parking lot, Autumn officially became my first girlfriend. We started spending a lot of time together. During the show, we made goo-goo eyes at each other whenever we had the chance.

There was just one problem—I had an extreme case of internalized homophobia. I wasn't ready to be "out." I was concerned what the other Rockettes would think. After all, we share a dressing room. I see them naked. They might think I'm looking at them in a sexual way. Yes, it is partly my own paranoia. So often, however, perhaps out of ignorance and fear, people assume that if you're gay, then you're automatically attracted to any person of the same sex.

The Rockette dressing rooms are on one side of the stage and the dancer/singer dressing rooms are on the opposite side. I live a double life within the parameters of the theatre. On my side of the dressing room, I never mention Autumn's name. *Autumn who? Oh, yes, Autumn, that's my favorite season.* When I make my way, as inconspicuously as possible, over to Autumn's dressing room, poof, I'm a lesbian, giving her little pecks on the lips and hugs before shows.

The reason for my split behavioral state is my level of comfort. The dancers and singers in the show are not as prissy or uptight as some of the Rockettes. Many of the Rockettes behave as gracefully outside of shows as they do onstage. The dancers and singers, and now me by association with Autumn, let our hair down a bit more. We actually associate with the stagehands. We party together after shows, smoke a little bud, occasionally snort a line or two of coke, and, of course, drink a lot. From a social perspective, I see the Rockettes as the conservatives and the dancers/singers as the liberals. Between my internalized homophobia and the air of poised conceit that floats through the Rockette dressing room, I decide I'd better keep Autumn a secret.

Autumn doesn't understand why one minute I'm into her and the next minute I'm ignoring her. Eventually, she grows sick of it and breaks up with me. But I can't stay away from her. By the end of the season, I decide I am moving back to New York City because Autumn lives there. I think that by moving to the liberal island of Manhattan, I'll be able to ditch my conservative Bible Belt of Branson homophobic fears.

The Great Divide

From the time I prematurely popped out of my mother's womb, the stage was set for me to become a dancer. My mother had been taking dance lessons for years, and so, naturally, when I turned three, she enrolled me in my first tap and ballet class. Once a week, on Saturdays, Mommy would take me to my dance class, where I'd stand in front of the mirror, proudly dressed in my black leotard and pink ballet tights, learning how to point and flex my feet, shuffle-ball-change, pirouette, and self-critique for the first time.

I absolutely fell in love with dance. By the way that my teacher, Ms. Nina, praised me with her endearing glances, showering me with attention, I knew that dance was my special gift. Almost immediately, dance defined me. Even in elementary school, my friends knew me as Greta, the dancer.

As my skill level increased, so did my dance class load. Soon, I was taking classes three days a week, after which, I'd sit inside the studio, along the back wall, watching my mother's dance classes. I would keep one eye on my homework and the other on Mommy's high kicks. All of the dancers at the studio commented on

Mommy's beautiful long legs. I aspired to dance as gracefully as my mother. I could tell that we shared the same adoration for dance by the way her spirit lit up each time her body became one with the music. Eventually, Mommy and I were spending four or five days a week at the studio.

Daddy, on the other hand, did not share our love for dance. In fact, my impression as a child is that he hated dance. I think he saw dance and my mother as the wedge that separated him from me and our otherwise perfect relationship. I felt this division between us early on, unsure how to create a blissful balance.

As a child, I felt like Daddy's little girl. He was charismatic, fun, loving, and playful, and always making jokes. Early on, he took me to the golf course, bowling, and attended my softball games (where I'd run away from the ball). Before school, he'd take me to Mr. D's donut shop. I always felt that he wanted to be in my life and make me happy. On the weekends, we'd watch our favorite reruns, like *Three's Company, M*A*S*H, Leave It to Beaver*, and *Make Room for Daddy*.

As an only child, the dynamic between my mother and father was difficult for me to balance. I felt badly for my mother because we both loved to dance. She just wanted to develop my talent. She didn't deserve my dad's growls toward her. At the same time, Daddy felt left out, so I felt bad about that, too. To ease his feelings of abandonment, I tried to learn softball and had my dad teach me how to hit golf balls at the driving range. It never lasted too long. Dance was always front and center. His resentment crowded any room that could be made for him.

Our family dynamic was prickly. My mom and dad coexisted as strangers. They were like two nasty neighbors fighting about the two inches of property line where the white picket fence sat. To some extent, we acted as mechanical robots without needs. On most days, we paraded around the house spouting off the usual one-liners from our list of empty discussion topics—our two favorites were weather and restaurant choices. In truth, though, we each had needs that were not being met. And we hadn't any clue as to how to address them.

My mother and father's conflictive relationship and deafening screaming wars worsened the more committed I became to dancing. There were fights about how much money dance cost (*"What a rip off dance classes are!"*) and fights about how much time dance took up in our lives. Growing up, I couldn't understand why my father made sarcastic snarls about Ms. Nina, the Old Bag, or why he rolled his eyes at Mommy practicing her tap routine in the kitchen. He'd shout, "Gayle, quiet! I'm watching television!" Everyone else appreciated her talent so much, why didn't he? For reasons I couldn't fathom at the time, he just didn't like dance.

Our family consisted of two teams swiftly moving in opposition, and I didn't know how to juggle their polarizing emotions. I loved dance. I loved Mommy. I loved Daddy. But, they didn't love each other. I felt guilty for not being able to help my mom when she was crying in our guest bathroom. I felt helpless when I saw in my father's eyes sadness and contempt for my mom. I felt angry that they wouldn't just grow up and get along.

Often, I'd try to convince my father to join my mother and me at the studio. After all, we wanted him there. I wanted us to be that picture-perfect family.

"Daddy," I'd say, trying to unglue his eyes from the television. "Why don't you come watch me take class? It's a lot of fun!"

"Uh . . . no," he'd say, sarcastically. "Why would I want to do that? Dance is so boring."

Boring? It was the love of my life!

"C'mon, Daddy. Pleeeease! I want you to come."

"Greta, I watch you dance. I come to your dance recitals."

"Okay," I'd say, scuttling off to class. *When I'm good enough*, I'd say to myself, *then he'll want to come watch me dance.*

For a long time, I thought that we were a normal family. Yes, my parents fought, but didn't all parents fight? Both of my parents held great jobs; my father was in management at an insurance company, and my mother was in finance at an international engineering firm. They'd go to the gym together (although they took separate cars), and dressed up for Halloween in matching 1980s rocker costumes. My dad bought my mom a nice fur coat for Christmas. The three of us went out to dinner as a family several times a week. We'd regularly watch movies together. And we ate Sunday dinners at home.

In the elegantly sculpted space between the impeccably dressed walls of our family home, however, a subtle yet raw bitterness prevailed. My parents didn't talk to one another, they shouted. Many nights, I'd hide underneath my bedcovers, my hands clutched to my ears, trying vainly to block out the nightly verbal money battles that raged in our kitchen. Before bed, I would strategically position my Cabbage Patch Kid dolls and other stuffed animals to shield me from my fears, hoping that when I woke up, my parents would magically be happy.

On the outside, we attempted to look happy. But even the strained smiles on my parent's faces in our family photos provide insight into our darker reality. Each of us suffered in our own way. My father used Southern Comfort to deaden the pain of his reality. My mom was a compulsive cleaner, and would come unglued if the furniture moved off its mark or if a rug wasn't in its assigned spot on the kitchen floor.

My parents also obsessed a lot about food and weight. There were diet pills in dresser drawers, weight-loss gadgets, and exercise equipment in our house. My dad ran miles in the hot sun in a sweat-provoking silver plastic garbage bag suit. (I often worried that he would drop dead from heat exhaustion.) My mom was regularly drinking Slim-Fast or eating Lean Cuisine. Their diet was one more way to shift focus off their real problems.

As a child, I didn't have the coping skills on which my parents relied. My anxiety came out mostly in the form of migraine headaches. From a psychoanalytic perspective, my chronic ear infections might leave an analyst to wonder what I didn't want to hear. I constantly walked on eggshells, doing my best not to let their sharp shells of resentment puncture my heels.

I tried to be the buffer. If I was the best that I could be, I hoped we could be happy again. Once, when my mom saw me crying, she said, "Greta, when I'm unhappy, I just put on some lipstick and I become happier." Unlike my father, whose anger for my mother was apparent, my mother lived in a sort of ignorance-is-bliss denial bubble. The lines of hurt and rage in her eyebrows, now erased by Botox, provide more accurate insight. Even the spectacular shade of Rockette Red lipstick couldn't cover up our unhappiness.

I wanted to believe we were happy. I'd boast to my friends how wonderful our lives were. *My mom is such an amazing cook. My dad is the best golfer and bowler. Our house is perfectly decorated. My mom takes me shopping every weekend. We go out for dinner almost every night of the week. I've never heard the words, "We can't afford that."*

My parents never hugged or kissed each other. They never gazed into each other's eyes and smiled. I never heard either one of them say to the other, "I love you." Never. They had a hard enough time saying it to me. The closest we felt to happy was when we ate dinner out. Food was our one common love.

WHEN I WAS thirteen, Mommy and I decided that if I wanted to dance professionally—which was exactly what I wanted to do—then I'd need to advance my training. Ms. Nina's studio was for dancers who wanted to dance "just for fun," as if dancing was just another extracurricular activity, like Girl Scouts or the school choir. Mommy knew dance was my life, and so we started surveying other studios that were more in the public eye of Kansas City.

After visiting a few studios around town, I enrolled at Dixie Bell Dance Center, which was located about five minutes from my house in Shawnee, Kansas. The dancers at this center were serious about dance. A select group of them performed throughout the year in regional competitions, local parades, and holiday events. Dixie Bell dancers were easily identifiable. They pranced around town wearing shiny green and black jackets that read, *The Kansas City Tap and Jazz Troupe.* I wanted to be a part of such an exclusive group. I wanted to wear a fancy jacket. *Then, I'd really be something special.*

Every fall, Dixie Bell held auditions for the dance troupe. I was determined to be a part of this exceptional clique. My audition was stellar. Several weeks later, after I received my very own green and black jacket, with my name monogrammed on the front left corner, I sat on my bed and thought to myself, *This is just the beginning of future successes.* Yep, I was going places. Places that extended far past our affluent Johnson County, Kansas, state line.

By the end of the year, our dance troupe had qualified for the National Showstopper Dance Competition, which meant that we were going to California. For weeks, we held fundraisers, we sold M&M's at grocery stores, held bake sales at school, and washed cars at fast food chains, strutting around in our bikinis and boxer shorts, trying to lure drivers to let us squeegee their windows and scrub their wheel wells.

We eventually did raise enough money. For a week, we gallivanted around Los Angeles, putting our hands and feet in the celebrity cement prints at Grauman's Chinese Theatre and taking our photographs with Mickey Mouse at Disneyland.

On the last day of our trip, my mom bought me an outfit at one of the fancy boutiques along Rodeo Drive. Mommy's happy. I'm happy. Somehow, the whole world seemed happier. It's amazing how spending money lifts one's spirits.

"Now, Greta," my mother said, leaving the store. "Let's not tell your father about this, okay?"

"Oh, I won't," I assured her, remembering times when we'd kept bags from other shopping trips locked in my mother's trunk. I knew that this wasn't the first secret and probably would not be the last one we'd keep from Daddy.

The next morning, we drove to LAX airport. My mom called my father to see when he was going to pick us up. While on the phone with him, worry forced the skin on my mother's forehead to scrunch. Her lips glued shut with anger.

"What's wrong, Mommy?"

"Your father says he's not coming to pick us up at the airport."

"Why? What do you mean he's not coming? How will we get home from the airport?"

"He just decided, Greta. He's not picking us up. We have to take a bus, and then he's going to pick us up from the Ramada Inn by our house."

I didn't understand. *Doesn't he want to see us? Doesn't he want to see me, and hear all about my Hollywood adventures?*

Shortly after Mommy and I arrived in Kansas City, we hopped on the Super Shuttle bus, with other travelers whose loved ones didn't want to pick them up either. The bus dropped us off in the circle drive of the Ramada Inn. Mommy and I waited by the curb. It was a hot summer morning and we were tired. We waited in silence, our minds distracted by our own narratives.

"Mommy," I asked, at one point. "Why do you think Daddy doesn't want to come pick us up?"

"I don't know, Greta. Probably because he's mad at me for some reason." *He's always mad at you. I hate it when he's mad at you.*

Mommy's eyes held a level of sadness that she usually covered up with false cheerfulness.

"I'm sure he'll be coming soon, though."

"Okay, Mommy." I put my head on my suitcase to rest it for a moment. *I hope Daddy's in a better mood when he picks us up. I can tell him about my trip and how well I danced. That should help.* I didn't really believe my thoughts, but I could try.

After what seemed like forever, my dad pulled into the circle drive. The car barked at us with its horn, our signal to hurry up and climb in the car.

"Hi, Daddy!" I chimed, once inside the car, hoping to snap him out of whatever was bothering him.

"Hi. How was your trip?" His tone was terse and flat. He didn't look at or say anything to Mommy. He'd turned into our chauffer, directed by his boss to wear his best poker face and never say a word.

I started telling him all about the competition, and the trophies we won, chattering on like white noise. I could see in the rearview mirror my father's eyes filled with years of built-up resentment. Soon, I stopped rambling. *Just shut up, Greta, it's not helping.* For the rest of the ride we drove in silence. I stared out the window, wondering how I would cheer my dad up later. I loved making him laugh. He was so funny. But this, this was not funny.

That moment, I realized our family was in big trouble. We were falling apart. My mom and dad had outgrown the costumes they wore for their parts of devoted husband and wife. They had no more masks to cover their raw bitter emotions. It wasn't like the costumes my mother had sewn for me, where she could add a dart here, or put a new zipper there. There was no fixing this. Our family had permanent damage.

Dancing into Destruction

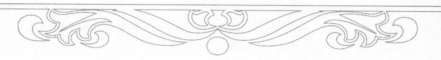

E ating disorders danced around the edges of my life for several months before actually taking a whopping leap to front and center. Between eighth grade and freshman year of high school, my eyes and ears awoke to a new world. Suddenly, and seemingly for the first time, I was seeing extreme thinness and hearing chatter of eating disorders everywhere.

"Ladies, today we are going to discuss eating disorders. When I was younger, in the ballet world, I was anorexic," Linda, my ballet teacher, began. To me, she still looked anorexic, so I can't imagine what she looked like years ago.

"Anorexia is very dangerous, and you all are beautiful the way you are." Linda continued for twenty more minutes, but I wasn't paying attention. I was fantasizing. I was one of her favorite students, and felt that if I became anorexic, then she would love me even more. This was my golden ticket. Earlier in the year, I had tried Slim-Fast, like my mom was doing. While she obsessed about her own weight, she always told me I didn't need to lose weight. *Greta, you have such muscular arms.* That never worked for me. I felt I had the shoulders of a linebacker.

I wasn't satisfied. I noticed that Linda always ate Special K and fat-free yogurt in a large Dannon container. I tried to exist on fat-fee yogurt and Special K, like I saw her eat daily, but I never had the discipline. I'd do it for a few days, but then gave in to eating Mexican or Chinese food with my parents.

Around this time, I also became best friends with a girl named Alyssa who lived around the corner. We instantly hit it off when she and her younger siblings handed me paper towels for the mint-chip ice cream dripping down my arm while walking past their house. The first time I came to Alyssa's house, her mother had just been released from the hospital. Her mom was the first person I knew who had been hospitalized for an eating disorder.

Alyssa's mom had brought home a Taco Bell salad. I didn't know it was her first meal out of the hospital. All I knew was that I liked Taco Bell. Especially its buttery fried taco shell. As Alyssa's mom began to eat, she could feel us hovering like beady-eyed vultures. In a split second she went from calm to enraged, screaming, "Just eat it! Eat the salad!!" before storming off to her bedroom. Frightened by her dramatic performance, I made my exit. Of course, I snatched a piece of the taco shell for the short walk home.

After that first encounter, I became extremely close with Alyssa's family. I was kind of obsessed with Alyssa's mom. I learned a lot about eating disorders, and I started to share with her about my blossoming disordered eating. She warned me, "Greta, don't mess with eating disorders. You will think you are in control, but it will control you."

I didn't believe her.

Alyssa's mom gave me that parental hit of affection I was looking for every time I went to her house. I'd watch television in her bed, lying beside her as if she were my human pillow. Their house was totally different than ours. It wasn't tidy and it was filled with kids.

Sometimes after spending the night, I'd leave with a stomachache because I didn't want to use the toilet that Alyssa's younger brother had pissed all over. Still, I loved it. The best part was that they talked about feelings and showed affection. There was no covert implication on how someone should be. Even if they lived in chaos, they were free to just be themselves.

I WAS ABOUT to start high school and was excited that I had been chosen for the freshman cheerleading squad. Many on my squad talked obsessively about losing weight. I noticed how skinny and pretty many of them were compared to me. I wished I could be waif-like instead of muscular. In the hallways at school, rumors swirled about a girl who lost a drastic amount of weight during the summer. *Can you believe how much weight she's lost? I think she's anorexic.* A normal reaction for me would've been to feel the same look of disgust and sadness these kids' faces showed while looking at this incredibly shrinking girl. When I looked at her, however, I felt envious. I wanted to be that special. I wanted to have that much control and discipline.

During my first year—in my health class of all places—I learned how to throw up. We were watching, *Kate's Secret,* a Meredith Baxter Birney movie about a young bulimic woman. I wavered between disgust and fascination. I watched Kate sit on the floor of a grocery store shoving Twinkies into her mouth, Twinkies that later resurfaced in her bathroom toilet. By the end of the movie, I'd come to a conclusion: throwing up could be a viable solution to my dieting woes. It was in that moment that the thought came to me: *I'm going to see if I can make myself throw up, just for fun.* Any experiment to help me lose weight, to open up the endless possibilities for attention, fulfillment, and happiness, gave me a jolt.

The following year, I began studying at Danceworks Conservatory. During my audition for enrollment, the ballet teacher told me I was too old to make it as a dancer. They awarded me a partial scholarship anyway because, despite my old age, I had natural talent. I traveled thirty minutes each way to take four hours of classes, five days a week. I worked hard in class, determined to prove my ballet mistress' projections about my dance career wrong.

In early fall, my school held the annual meet-and-greet cheerleading banquet for all of the parents and cheerleaders to meet one another. The night of the event was a cool October evening, that glorious time of year when tree leaves are beautiful shades of orange and brown. Less than an hour before the banquet, my parents, as usual, were yelling at each other in the kitchen. Over the years, I had learned to ignore their fights, but on this night, I couldn't. As I stood in front of my bedroom mirror analyzing my appearance and trying to block out the sound of their familiar shouting, my father confirmed my worst fears.

"After the banquet, I'm out of here."

What? He didn't say that. He couldn't have said that. Did he say he was leaving?

A stinging sensation of anxiety stabbed my chest, and I couldn't move. In the middle of my bedroom, I stood paralyzed, frozen with fear and disbelief that my father was actually leaving.

The slam of the garage door shook my body, and I ran downstairs to my mother.

"Is he really leaving?" I asked my mother in a panic.

My mother sat at our kitchen table, casually flipping through a magazine, looking as if she was thinking about the weather or scrolling down her mental list of things to do.

"No, Greta. He just needs some time to cool down. He's not really leaving."

My gut told me that she was lying to herself and to me.

"Don't worry. I'm sure he's coming home. He just wanted to drive separately to let off some steam. Are you ready to leave for the banquet?"

Banquet? Who wants to go to a banquet at a time like this? Fuck the banquet, I want to say. Instead, I reply, "Yeah, I'm ready."

We drive to the banquet in silence, our heads continually replaying the scene at home. Funneling around my mind were questions I couldn't answer. Will we have to move out of our house? When will I see my father? Who will take care of us? I tried to focus on something else.

Staring outside my window, I admired the display of Halloween witches and cobwebs that draped the front doors of the houses in my neighborhood. As I looked, I could feel the chilly air of the nearing winter clinging to the car window, trying to inch its way in, as it always does, just before the changing of the seasons. I couldn't help thinking that my parents and I were approaching a season of change, too—a season I didn't recognize. A season that I was sure was bringing unpredictable weather.

As we entered the banquet, my eyes darted from corner to corner in search of my father. There across the room, I spotted him talking to my aunt. For a moment, I felt relief that he was still in my presence. I resisted joining my dad and aunt because I was afraid that I would cry and scream and reveal his secret that he was abandoning my mother and me. My mother and I mingled with the other parents and cheerleaders, wearing our happy faces of denial. I scanned the room, noticing the joy that painted the faces of the huddles of PTA moms and cheerleaders. I wanted to feel what they felt. As I glanced over at my father once more, I could see that he too was trying to deny reality. His face appeared so at ease that I thought he may have changed his mind. Maybe he wasn't angry with my mother anymore. I hoped so. Somewhere inside me, I knew the truth. My mom, my dad, and I were acting; publically performing as a family one last time.

A few minutes later, I scoped the room and realized that my father had left. He didn't say goodbye, he just left. Relief left me, panic ensued, and I needed to escape. Immediately, I told my mother that I wanted to leave. She was in midconversation, but I didn't care. Her eyebrows frowned at me with their familiar shape of irritation.

"In a minute, Greta," she replied.

Twenty minutes later, I walked into the house and headed straight to my mom and dad's closet. Gone. The white wire hangers on which an array of golf and business shirts used to hang now lay naked and abandoned. I felt like Joan Crawford in *Mommie Dearest*. I felt like I was standing still and the room was spinning, the wire hangers slapping me across the face. I wanted to crumple in a pile on the floor and cry like a baby like Joan did. I, too, felt out of control. Only my rage and anguish was different.

Until this moment, I believed there was still a chance that he was not going to follow through with his plans. As I looked at the newly vacant space, I could feel my heart pounding through my chest. My world was crumbling. I wanted to collapse onto the floor, sick with emotion. Instead, I refrained, pulled myself together, dusted myself off with the palms of my hands, and paraded into the kitchen to attack the only target available: my mom.

"See, I told you he was leaving! You said he wasn't, but I knew he was! How long is he going to be gone for?"

My mother didn't want to tell me that he was gone forever, and so she replied the only way she knew how. "Well, Greta, I don't know how long he'll be gone for, but I'm sure he'll be back."

"But he didn't even call me! When is he going to call me?" I wanted answers that my mother was unable to provide.

"I don't know, Greta," she said, "but I'm sure he'll call soon."

Later that evening, my father called.

"Daddy, when are you coming home?" I could hear the sadness in his voice.

"Greta, I'm not sure." This was not helpful. I needed to know right that minute. I could feel my tension building and my reservoir of tears approaching flood level.

"Well, is it going to be a week? A month? Three months?"

He replied with practically the same answer. "Greta, I just don't know."

After we hung up, I needed someone to run and cry to, but there was no one. My mother stood right in front of me, but I couldn't run to her. We didn't hug, touch, or discuss feelings. In her presence, I was only allowed to feel happiness. There was no room for conflicting feelings. I raced upstairs to my bedroom, unable to push down my feelings any longer. Once alone in the privacy of my bedroom, the dam broke, and my reservoir of tears poured out of me. It was a cold night. I lay awake in my bed bundled beneath layers of blankets, sobbing for hours about the uncertainty of my future, until I finally fell asleep.

A few days later, my father called to tell me that he wasn't coming home. We were officially on separate teams. Soon after, my mother filed for divorce. *Divorce? No one in my family divorces. We are Catholic for Christ's sake.*

SHORTLY AFTER MY parents' separation, my dad took me to an amusement park, World's of Fun. *The irony.* I couldn't imagine having to spend all day riding roller coasters with him. Riding in the car, I felt like I didn't know this newly single dad, inhabiting a bare apartment, decorated with a lone couch and large flat-screen television. Where was the Daddy who threw softballs to me in the backyard, who I laid with watching TV on the couch? My dad sensed this, I think, by my forty-five minutes of silence during the drive. My dad parked the car, but then hesitated before getting out.

"Greta?" he said. "How are you doing?" He had never asked me that in this tone. There wasn't a need before.

"Okay," I said, my eyes on the carpet floor mat.

"I just want you to know . . . that it's not your fault that I left." Tears rose to the surface.

"I know," I said. I know it isn't really my fault, but I've always thought that if I could've done something better, then maybe . . . .

My dad started to cry. This broke my heart. "Greta, I just want you to know that . . . that I love you."

"I love you, too," I said. Months of tears I'd been keeping inside poured out of me. My dad grabbed me and gave me a big hug. We were both still crying as we embraced.

A few minutes later, we got out of the car to start our theme park adventure. For the first time, I felt like we were going to be okay. It was the first time in months that I felt safe. During our day, we sipped lemonade, snacked on pizza, and rode roller coasters. The theme park lived up to its name. For a day, I lived in a world of fun.

EVEN THOUGH BOTH of my parents told me their separation was not my fault, I became very depressed. I didn't show it in my emotions, but I couldn't care less about my appearance and would rather wear pajama pants than dress up for school. I had no control or choice of what was happening. I dazed off in my classes, my mind lost in uncertainty. "Greta, are you with us?" my teacher would say. *Fuck school. For that matter, fuck my life.* I couldn't see what was ahead for me. I needed something to stabilize the uncertainty.

During this time, *Kate's Secret* from my freshman year health class entered my mind. Kate wouldn't be the only one with secrets. Keeping secrets was something I was good at by this time, and I was ready to have something private of my own.

I didn't connect the emotional dots. I didn't realize then that the decision I was about to make would change the course of my life forever. The eating disorder was about to grab the starring role of my life.

On the pivotal day, I methodically walk into my house, drop my backpack onto its usual dumping ground, the couch, and flip on the television. Besides dancing, television is my favorite pastime. My entire life, I've been a rerun junkie. Every day after school, I escape into the lives of Marsha Brady, Jack Tripper, and Beaver Cleaver, knowing so much about each of them that I can predict their next moves.

I kick off my shoes and mosey over to the kitchen, feeling the smooth ceramic tile underneath my athletic socks, as I pirouette and jeté my way beside the kitchen counter. Before I open the kitchen cabinets, I know exactly what I will see: Skippy Peanut Butter, Triscuit crackers, Lorna Doone cookies, and an assortment of low-calorie snacks. *Yuck.* Still, I open the glossy oak doors in hopes that a treat of some sort, one that may have been hiding up to this point, will materialize. I inspect both shelves. Just as I predicted, the same foods sit in their designated spots. Each name-brand snack screams, "Pick me! Pick me!" as I look at them. I start with four or five Lorna Doone cookies. I open the box of Triscuits. *I hate Triscuits.* I dip a couple of the roughly textured wheat crackers into a thick glob of peanut butter to try to make me forget how much I despise these salty, sandpaper squares. I want something different and exciting. As if such an item exists in my parents' kitchen cabinets.

On the second shelf, I cram my hand in between the requisite stash of seasonal edible gifts that have been living in our cabinets for at least five years, but which still remain, because we, for whatever reason, have yet to throw them away. These are the gifts given to my mother by acquaintances like our neighbors or her coworkers, gifts that dwell, I think, in everyone's kitchen cabinets from time to time. The beautifully wrapped jars and boxes that she receives from people who don't really know her, because if they did, they would know that she would never eat a fruitcake.

After finding nothing but a bag of chocolate espresso balls, I move toward the refrigerator. My palate waters, as I hear the familiar suction when opening the refrigerator and freezer doors, knowing that my odds of finding something exciting in the various compartments are much greater. I tease my tongue with a few pieces of Monterey Jack cheese, before making my way to what I hope will be the jackpot. A warm and fuzzy sensation, like opening presents on Christmas morning, surrounds me.

When I see it, excitement radiates throughout my body. I reach in and take hold of it with both hands. I extend the cardboard container filled with Jeno's pepperoni pizza in front of me, and admire the bits of heavily processed pepperoni, cheese, and crunchy crust pictured on the box. A triumphant blare of trumpets sounds in the background. I imagine a short, balding tub of a man standing behind a podium in an arena grabbing a microphone with one hand and a pizza box with the other, holding it up to the crowd and announcing, "*We have a winner! We have a winner!*" The crowd roars.

I can barely wait for the oven to preheat. I want it now. My hands invade the box of Lorna Doone cookies again, this time grabbing three or four. Ten minutes later, I hear the timer on the oven shout, signaling that it's time to put my pizza in. Impatiently, I wait for the pepperoni to brown and my crust to crisp, trying hard to zone out to the television while it cooks.

Finally, the aroma of melted cheese lingers in the air, letting me know my pizza is ready. Before I open the oven door, I can hear the sizzle of the pepperonis as they spit, pleading for cool air. My little pie of heaven is ready. After taking my pizza out of the oven, I cut it into six symmetrical slices, making sure an equal amount of pepperonis and cheese top each piece. I balance my almost-too-hot-to-touch pizza with the tips of my fingers, bringing it so close to my face that the aroma slithers up my nose. Just when I'm about to sink my teeth into the meticulously chosen first slice, I force myself to stop. I'm not going to burn the roof of my mouth like I do almost every other day I eat pizza. Not knowing what else to do, I sit and stare at the pizza. If I stare at it long enough, it's bound to cool down.

I take the first bite. The combination of sauce and fat effortlessly slides down my throat. *Pure ecstasy. Ah, yes, the feeling I've been waiting for.* I shove each bite a little faster into my mouth and try to recapture the pleasure that only the first bite can bring. As I eat my pizza, I can't help but think about the actions that will follow my eating. Like most people, I've always hated throwing up. *I wonder if it's going to be every bit as awful as being truly sick.* Nearing the last bite, excitement overrides the sadness that usually hangs over my head when finishing a meal. I'll soon be undertaking a new task.

Typically, I run up the steep flight of stairs to the second floor, but today I saunter casually, walking upward in a slow march, deliberating with each step whether I should follow through with my plans. A few more strides place me inside my bathroom. The cold white tile chills the bottom of my feet. The familiar coral towels hang neatly on their racks. The tub and toilet have their usual gloss from the weekly Sunday bleaching. Still, the bathroom looks completely different to me. I'm about to enter into an unfamiliar realm, which I feel like I've been preparing to enter for years.

I'm face to face with the toilet. My body sways back and forth with apprehension. *Why are you doing this? You know this is wrong.* I contemplate "this" for a few more minutes, thinking about what all of "this" will mean when I've completed the dirty deed. *There are other ways to lose weight. All you have to do is have some discipline and eat healthy. Just turn away.* I feel torn. I walk forward on a tightrope of sanity, trying to decide whether I want to keep the delicate balance or free fall into the irrational, unclear if there's a safety net below.

Denial taunts my brain, *Go on, Greta, just do it!* My rational side knows that anyone who would even consider this behavior is in some respect crazy, but I decide to pay that side no attention. *What else do you have to lose? You hate school, you feel ugly, and your parents are getting a divorce.* The deal is sealed.

I stand hip-width apart facing the toilet, lean over, and put my hand inside my mouth. I immediately realize that I have never been this close to the bacteria-infested waters of a toilet. I can see my reflection in the water, confused eyes staring back at me. As I hang upside down, I can't help but notice the superb job my mother has done cleaning the toilet. Spotless. I've never appreciated my mother's cleaning ability more than I do at this moment.

My fingers are like foreign objects to my throat and I can taste the combination of greasy pizza and salt residue on the back of my tongue. I inch my fingers further back in my throat until my gag reflex engages. *Not much is happening.* I shove my hand in harder, my eyes begin to tear and I start to cough, but nothing else. *I don't understand. This isn't what happened in the movie. Kate simply leaned over and out it came.* Part of me wants to give up, but the other part of me is on a mission. Now desperate to produce any evidence of pizza in the toilet, I decide to try harder. *Focus, Greta!*

Once again, I hunch over and shove my fingers down my throat as hard as I can. My gag reflex finally grows sick of fighting with my fingers, and soon I can feel rough edges of crust and pepperoni moving fast in reverse digestion. I'm surprised that the food tastes the same, a definite plus. As the food exits my mouth and dives into the toilet, the water rebounds. Splatters of water and pizza hit my face. The grossness of it all doesn't faze me. *My mission was a success.*

A flush of the toilet disposes the evidence. I stare into my blood-shot eyes and look at my red face in the mirror, taking a moment to digest it all. A dichotomy of thoughts and emotions flood my brain as I try to assess the situation. I don't know if I should be afraid of myself or pat myself on the back. After a bit more deliberation, elation supersedes any earlier fear. I look into my eyes once more and smile. *A job well done, Greta.*

I threw up at least fifty times between that first afternoon and the day my parents' divorce was final. They already are dating the very people who eventually become my stepparents: Kent and Lavada. My mom knows about my bulimia because one of my dance teachers told her. When she found out, she was pissed. "Greta, you just have to stop!!" I agreed, of course, but was in too deep at that point. My father doesn't know, exactly, but knows something is different. He can't believe how much I eat.

"Greta, don't you think eating an entire cheesecake is a lot for you and your friend to eat?" he asks, laughing in disbelief.

"We were hungry, what can I say?"

After almost every meal, I immediately charge upstairs to my bathroom. My mother tries to deny my behavior, but sometimes, when Kent isn't around, she is fed up. Rightfully so. I can't imagine the terror in knowing you have a daughter who is trying to hurt herself. We have practically the same conversation every Sunday. It goes like this:

"Yum," I say, scraping the fork in between the grooves of my plate to scoop up any last fragments of food. "Good dinner, Mommy."

"Thanks, I'm glad you liked it." I hand her my plate to clean, as if she's my personal maid, and go over to the couch to sit down. My mom watches me as I wander into the living room and plop down onto the couch.

Since the beginning of dinner, I've been trying to calculate how long I'll have to sit here watching *60 Minutes* before I can excuse myself. I can feel my mother glaring at my nervousness as she puts away the dishes, and after a couple of minutes, I can no longer stand sitting in my skin.

"Well," I say. "I'm going upstairs to take a bath."

My mother asks, "Greta, why don't you stay down here with us and watch television? You hardly spend time with me and Kent." I'm pretty sure she knows that taking a bath is code for puking, but she wants to make this about me spending time with them.

"I know, but I really want to take a bath. I feel cold. I need to warm myself up."

"Cold? How can you feel cold? It's the middle of the summer!"

"You know me. I'm always cold." And with that, I race upstairs to the bathroom, turn the bath water on, and try to throw up as quietly as I can.

Other times, though, usually when Kent is out of town, she doesn't deny it. As soon as I turn the bathroom water on, she yells from the foot of the stairs, "I know that you're not taking a bath. God damn it, Greta! You're puking!"

Sometimes, I'll come out with a coral-colored towel wrapped around my body and take my hair out of my ponytail, as if my outfit will convince her. "I am, too! Look at me, I'm about to get in!"

In these times, I can't puke in the toilet. God forbid I ever keep a meal down. My other choices are the sink or the bathtub, which are never good options. The food clogs the drain, I become panicked, and then I have to scoop the clogged bits of food with my hands, transfer them into and flush the toilet, which is what I was trying to avoid doing in the first place.

During the summer, an incident occurs—The Spaghetti Incident—that makes it impossible for my mother to deny my behavior. I can't resist casserole-type meals, and after polishing off two platefuls of my mother's delicious spaghetti and meat sauce, I'm stuffed.

"I think I'll go organize my closet," I say. I wait for my mother's response. *No comments. She bought it.*

As I walk into my room, my eyes dart from my dresser to my

stereo. I quickly go down on my hands and knees to look beneath the bed. *I need to find something to throw up in.* Nothing! I begin digging my hands through a cardboard junk box in my closet. *This'll work,* I muse, grabbing a large white plastic cup from the box. I go to my stereo and turn on Celine Dion to muffle the sound of my stomach heaving. I put the cup on my blue carpet, lean over, and throw up. *Success.*

Unexpectedly, I hear my mother talking to someone outside. I walk over to the window. It's just our neighbor, Mr. Longhibler. I turn my attention back to the cup. I close my eyes for a second, hoping that when I reopen them, what I see will be gone. My eyes don't deceive. Squinting through the paper-thin cracks of my eyes, I can already see the disaster. The cup is no longer sitting upright. It has tipped over onto its side. *Oh, Shit!* A thirty-two-ounce pool of semi-digested spaghetti *avec sauce rouge* is seeping and soaking its erosive juices into my blue carpet. *Oh—My—God!!* I cover my mouth with my hand to silence it from screaming. There is no way I'm going to be able to talk myself out of this one. *C'mon, Greta, think! You have to do something fast!*

I drop to my knees and hurriedly pick up as many handfuls of the stomach-acid-laced spaghetti as I can, throwing them sloppily back into the cup. A huge red stain—mixed with miniscule pieces of pasta—corrupts the carpet. *You idiot!* I can't believe how stupid I am. *How the hell are you going to get away with this, Greta?* I'm royally fucked. A thought comes to mind. *I've been keeping my room a mess lately, so I'll just throw a towel over the stain. Maybe Mommy won't notice.*

The next day, I uncover the towel to reveal a permanent stain of spaghetti sauce red. Now would be a perfect time to call the execs over at Crayola. *"Excuse me, Mr. Crayola? Could you come as quickly as you can? I've discovered a new reddish hue that I'd like you to take a look at. It's called Spaghetti Sauce Red."*

I crouch down to the stain and take a big whiff. The stench of day-old puke has set in and it is not cute. I look a little closer and see pieces of pasta embedded in the fibers of the carpet. I feel like I'm in that *Leave It to Beaver* episode where Beaver throws the soft ball through the garage window. "Gee Wally," Beaver says, staring at the busted window. "What are we going to tell Dad?" What am I going to tell Mommy? I'm pretty sure that I won't be coming away with a nice mother-daughter talk and a life lesson when my mom discovers this stain.

I walk out of my room to Kent's office, grab the scissors, and begin to cut pieces of pasta out of the carpet. I stand up and move away from the stain to gain perspective. *Yes, it looks a little better.* I tilt my head, as if looking at it from a different angle will make it less noticeable. Still, I know that there's no way that I can get this past my mother. *Oh well, nothing I can do now.* I throw the towel back over the stain.

One week later, I hear shrieks coming from upstairs. It's my mother.

"Greta! Get up here!"

What does she want now?

"I'm watching television, can't I come up later?"

"No! Get up here *now*!

Uh-oh. Her voice tells me that I'm in trouble. I start my trek up the long flight of stairs, and as I get about halfway up, it dawns on me that she has unveiled the stain. There's nothing I can do.

I walk into my room to find my mother with the towel in her hand, standing over the crusty, stained carpet.

"Greta, look at this! Look at this stain! How did it get here?" Her eyes tell me that she doesn't want to know, that she doesn't want it to be true. I won't let them down.

"Well . . . uh . . . I was eating some leftover spaghetti the other day and I spilled the bowl on the floor."

"Greta, it smells like puke."

She smelled it?!

"No, it doesn't." Denial is my only recourse.

"Greta, what did you do? Just leaned over and puked all over the floor?" She's mortified.

"No, Mommy, of course not." I'm shocked. How can she think I would do something so idiotic? I don't remind myself that attempting to puke in a top-heavy cup wasn't such a brilliant idea.

I deny all claims until Mommy finally has to let it go. Before long, my mom transitions into her comfortable cleaning mode, bent down on all fours, scrubbing the red stain, as though cleaning up her emotionally disturbed daughter's puke is part of her cleaning ritual every weekend. Being the domestic virtuoso that Mommy is, she manages to scrub away any evidence of my unsettling, spaghetti-sauce-carpet-puking behavior. We will never talk about the Spaghetti Incident again.

FOR AS MUCH time as my mother and I spend together, you'd think that we would be one of those mother-daughter "best friend" pairs. Growing up, many of my friends had this type of relationship with their mothers. They confided in their mothers about everything; they cuddled up with their mothers on their beds and watched television; they cried to their mothers when a boy crushed their hearts, or when their friends stabbed them in the back; they sought advice from their mothers about shaving their legs or plucking their eyebrows; they talked to their mothers about getting their periods and asked questions about sex.

In short, they were able to talk, really talk, to their mothers. I craved and envied my friends' mother-daughter relationships, and didn't understand why I didn't have that.

My mother and I did a lot of talking—about my clothes ("You should never wear pleats, it accentuates the hips,"), about the weather

("Wow, it's such a sunny day, isn't it?"), about my food ("You don't need another hot dog!"), about her food ("All I eat is a single egg for breakfast!") about my face ("Greta, you're not leaving this house without foundation on your face . . . you have got to cover it up . . . I mean . . . it's just . . . embarrassing!")—but we never talked about anything of substance.

My mother and I never had the conversations about growing pangs that my friends had with their mothers. In fact, at sixteen, when I got my period, I made my best friend call my mother, as I was too embarrassed. Every month following, I'd sneak a box of Tampax into my mother's grocery cart, the way a chubby ten-year-old slyly sneaks a pack of M&M's in between the milk and apples at the checkout line while his mom flips through *People* magazine.

While, as a child, I couldn't name my feelings or know why I felt a certain way, I always remember feeling like something was missing between my mother and I. It wasn't that I questioned my mother's love. I knew by the way she bought me anything I wanted and helped me fulfill my dreams in dance that she loved me a great deal.

During the summers, from the time I was about two years old, my mother and I'd go to the neighborhood pool. The Prairie Village Pool was where my mother had been swimming since she was a little girl and, eventually, where she'd become a top swimmer. Like at the dance studio, everyone at the pool knew my mother, the talented diver. We have so many photos together of those summers at the pool: My mother and I sitting on our beach towels, in picture-perfect poses, with the Coppertone bottle in the background and my eyes squinting from the bright sun, waiting for Grandma Sally to snap the Polaroid.

One sweltering summer Sunday, when I was around five years old, my mom and I walked to the pool, just as we'd done many other Sundays.

"Greta," my mother said. "Hold my hand, we're about to cross the street."

I grabbed her hand and, immediately, a tinge of uneasiness flowed through me. I looked at the hand clutching mine, my eyes following the line up my mother's arm until I gazed at her face. Clearly, the person's hand I was holding onto was my mother's; but it felt strange. I wasn't used to a physical connection. Nervousness fluttered around my stomach with my awareness. *It must be me. When I'm a teenager, things will change. That's when mothers and daughter grow closer.* I didn't have a name for it yet, but years later I recognized it as a lack—lack of connection, lack of affection, lack of nurturing—on a deep emotional level.

What I identified then, as nervousness, was really the first feelings of the chronic emptiness and disconnection I felt with both of my parents, as well as in the world. I knew my parents loved me and would do anything for me, just because they were my parents. For some reason, though, I didn't feel the security of knowing that I'm not only their daughter but also a daughter who is special and worth something just as I am, without having to achieve anything or be good looking.

There were a few times when I was very young, however, that I remember lying on our couch with my eyes closed, so that my mother could tickle my face. I loved that. As I got older, though, the physical affection went from scarce to nonexistent. Besides the pats on the back masked as hugs given to me on birthdays or holidays, my mom wasn't capable, for some reason, of giving a motherly kiss or an empathetic touch. The emotional well was dry. To warrant an inkling of affection or compassion meant that I either had to achieve greatness or had to have fallen ill.

Perfection equals love. Sick equals love.

SHORTLY AFTER THE divorce, my maternal grandmother, Grandma Patty, and I had many conversations about my mother's discomfort with showing affection. Neither of us understood it.

"All I know," my Grandma once said, "is that when your mother turned sixteen years old, I came up from behind her to give her a big bear hug and wish her a happy birthday, and she just froze." For a split second, I felt a sense of sadness for my mother.

"I don't get it. Sherry, Pam, and Suzie aren't like that," I said, referring to my mother's younger sisters. "They're all very affectionate." My mother has three younger sisters, each of whom has several kids—all daughters. Sherry and Pam, second and third in birth order, are the PTA stay-at-home mom types. I imagine they had cookies waiting for my cousins as they arrived home from school. At holiday events, I closely watched the interactions between my aunts and my cousins. They never have any problems giving their children loving strokes of affection.

"I know, Greta, I know. I've tried to figure out why your mom doesn't open up. She's never been abused nor had anything ever happen to her. That's just the way she is. She's like her father."

"Well, it really sucks!" I replied, unsatisfied with her answer. I didn't want to hear that. I wanted her to tell me that, at some point, she will be able to show affection to me. She will be able to tell me, out loud—not through giving me money—that she is proud of me. She will hug me and reassure me that I am okay just as I am.

"I know, Greta. I've tried to talk to your mother, but I just can't crack her. The only thing she's told me is that she's a very complicated person. Your mother is just a different breed. But, you know, she loves you more than anything."

"I know," I quietly acknowledged. My mother has the best of intentions. At the same time, though, I am so confused. What is so hard about showing emotions? What is so hard about saying the words, "I love you," or, "I'm so proud of you"? Why is it so hard for my mother to physically touch me, yet she is quick to criticize? It's easier for her to judge than to love. I didn't get it. It felt unfair. *I just have to be better, somehow.*

DURING MY CHILDHOOD, Grandma Patty lived a few hours away at the Lake of the Ozarks, with my Grandpa Bob. After Grandpa Bob passed away, she moved back to Kansas City. Up to that point, I had spent most of my time with Grandma Sally, and didn't have the same level of closeness. Grandma Sally was more let loose than Grandma Patty, although, family holiday photos from when I was a baby, where they held drinks in one hand and a cigarette in the other, showed that they both liked to have a good time.

I was aware from a very young age that Grandma Patty had been in recovery from alcoholism for many years and was a religious Alcoholics Anonymous meeting maker. When I was about eight years old, I attended Grandma Patty's anniversary meeting to celebrate her milestone in sobriety, where Grandma Patty shared her story of recovery. Even back then, I was intrigued by the addictive cycle, asking, "Grandma Patty, were you *really* on a merry-go-round?"

My mom must have made Grandma Patty aware of my eating disorder, because her once general inquiries about me held a deeper connotation. She wanted to know *how* I was doing. After all, my parents were the first in our Catholic family to get divorced. And it wasn't like it was an amicable divorce.

"But Greta," she said one day, as she dropped me off at my house after we had eaten at our favorite hamburger joint. "Your parents are so much happier apart."

"But I'm not happy," I said.

"I know, Greta. I know you aren't." We hugged and kissed goodbye. I gave her a half-reassuring smile that I would be fine. I already knew where I was going. I wanted relief. I went into the house, straight up to my bathroom, and purged.

Grandma Patty and I were like two peas in a pod when it came to our addictive genes. She started hinting around that maybe a Twelve-Step Overeaters Anonymous program would help me.

"Greta," she said, on my eighteenth birthday, in her cheerful grandma voice. "I have a present for you."

Oh, goody, I think to myself. *I love presents.* Grandma Patty hands me a rectangular box. The perfect creases and folds of the metallic and hot pink paper tell me she had it wrapped at the seasonal kiosk at the mall that offers free gift wrapping. I undo the perfectly placed bow.

As soon as I remove the lid of the box, I see the book. I'm horrified. *The Twelve Steps and Twelve Traditions of Overeaters Anonymous.* What? Who's a compulsive overeater? Does she know anything? I'm a bulimic!

I cast a toothy performance smile over my fury and give Grandma Patty a quick "Thanks," but inside I'm about explode. She has some nerve. So what if she has twenty years of sobriety under her belt. Who does she think she is to bring me a book like this? Not to mention on my birthday, of all days!

I flip open to the first page. Grandma has written me a note. It reads, "To Greta, I love you very much." Ugh. I turn to the first chapter. "We Are Powerless Over Food and Our Lives Have Become Unmanageable." I'm disgusted. I know I've been bingeing and purging regularly for a while now, but I'm not powerless. I may feel out of control at times, but I have some power. And my life certainly is not unmanageable. *Unmanageable?* What does that even mean, anyway? It isn't as though I'm living under a bridge like some unfortunate drunk because I ate one too many gallons of ice cream. So I throw up a couple of times a day. Who cares? Everyone has an outlet. Besides, it doesn't interfere with my life that much. For the most part, my life is good.

It will be five years before I actually pick up that book again.

ONE YEAR AFTER my parents' divorce is finalized, I am in full-blown bulimia mode, bingeing and purging every day before dance class, and purging my dinner in the bathroom at the dance studio between my ballet and jazz classes. I'm taking diuretics, laxatives, diet pills, Ipecac syrup—shitting, shaking, and almost dying—and walk slyly past the school cafeteria workers with buttery homemade chocolate chip cookies stuffed in my jacket. I work in the school attendance office, where I forge letters signed by my mother, so I can binge and purge in solitude in my dark basement while watching the movie, *The Best Little Girl in the World*.

I cry to Alyssa's mom, "You were right, I am out of control." She listens to me, comforts me. She cares for me unconditionally and gives me attention. I think she has a conversation about my eating disorder with my mom and Kent.

Sick equals love.

ONE GREAT THING in my life was my dancing. During my junior year in high school, I moved up two levels in dance. Nicole, my ballet teacher, and Loren, my jazz teacher, noticed my talent.

While Nicole and Loren were both the current idols in my life, as a teen I was closer with Loren. She went out of her way to talk to me and ask questions about my life. I confessed my eating disorder to her, and she shared her past weight struggles with me. She told me how much she cared about me, and that I was a beautiful person regardless of the eating disorder. While I was never told to lose weight by my teachers, it always seemed like the ballerina waifs received most of the attention. At least, that was my perception.

Sick equals love. Thin equals love. Perfection equals love.

DURING MY JUNIOR year, I enrolled in what I thought would be a blow-off elective class, personal family relations. I had always been into psychology and, given the fucked up state of my family, I thought the class would be interesting. Mrs. Dinneen was the teacher. She was in her midforties with short blond hair. She also worked at the school where pregnant teenager girls go for their education. Between her empathy and my people-pleasing, we clicked instantly.

She quickly became another mentor in my life. I fantasized about her spending time with me, and nurturing my emptiness. I wanted her to see the depression. I wanted her to see that I wasn't okay. What was going on with me wasn't something a fresh coat of lipstick and a nice outfit would fix. I told her all about my eating disorder, and by the end of the year, I asked her if she would talk to my mom about it. Shortly thereafter, I started seeing my first therapist.

Loren, Nicole, and Mrs. Dinneen weren't the first teachers I tried to gain attention and affection from. I had been replaying this scene out with other teachers long before my eating disorder began. When I was in the first grade, I cried and cried on the first day at my new school, surrounded by unfamiliar faces.

"Don't cry, honey," Mrs. Lohmeyer, my new teacher, said, attempting to reassure me. "It'll be alright." Mrs. Lohmeyer was a tall middle-aged woman. Well, I was six years old, so middle-aged could mean she was twenty-five. She had short, thick, dark brown hair, with matching dark brown eyes. She paid attention to my tears, bending down and giving me a little hug before she went back to teaching. Her comforting words warmed my heart.

From that day forward, I latched onto her soft eyes and tender touch the way a bloodsucking leech clings to a twelve-year-old's leg in a dirty pond. For over a month, I cried daily, complaining of ear infections or other ailments, hoping to capture Mrs. Lohmeyer's attention. *Sick equals love.*

Repeatedly, she comforted me. I wanted more. Always. I tried further to win her over by being the perfect student. It worked. I was one of her favorites.

Perfection equals love.

In second grade, there was an incident where a pole fell on my head, which left me with a big knot. My teacher, Mrs. Player, comforted me as I sat in the classroom crying with an ice pack on my head. Whereas the year before, I wasn't conscious of my needs; by the time this happened, I specifically remember the feeling of wanting and trying to gain her attention, as well as the feeling of loss when I didn't get it. This was also probably the first time I felt feelings of associated shame.

Through the years, the list of teachers—and eventually therapists—I sought out grew, as did my hunger for a needed hit of heartfelt affection. As soon as a teacher or one of my friends' mothers gave me a morsel of affection, perhaps a stroke on my forearm or an empathetic squeeze, I'd be reminded of the physical affection that I craved but couldn't get, and whom I needed it from. The more attention these authority figures gave me, the more attention I craved, the more I felt I needed to perform, and the emptier I felt when their emotional wells went dry. Their nurturing touch and gentle words began to hurt, triggering stinging questions I tried to answer as to why my own mother couldn't give me the love that others so freely gave away. *What was wrong with me? What was so hard about showing me affection?* I didn't have the answers. I found myself in a double bind because that which I craved became the greatest source of my pain. I didn't know how to unleash myself from its gnawing grips.

All I knew was that I was hungry, very hungry.

Behind the Curtain

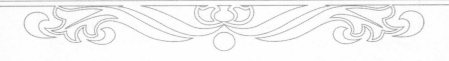

After quitting the underground world as a marijuana delivery girl, I prepare myself for the *All My Children* television debut. The summer speeds by, full of success. I don't live at the Markle Residence anymore. After a two-day session of constant bingeing in the Markle's television room, I had a mental break. I called my friend Stacey, one of Michele's class assistants, and admitted my behavior. Stacey told me to come over to her place in Queens as soon as I could. Now, I'm living with Stacey and three other dancers, Mara, Michelle, and Jenny.

Besides wanting to dance at the Music Hall and make Broadway Dance Center my second home, my other motivation for moving to New York was to date Autumn, my first real girlfriend.

Looking back now, I can hardly call it dating. We met up several times and had sex. The overriding shame I felt caused me to cancel several of our dates, and she eventually grew sick of it. The final time I asked her to meet up, I had decided that I was going to give up my internalized homophobia. Unfortunately, I'd canceled one too many times. She did agree to meet, but then she stood me up. No biggie. I binged on a Boston cream pie instead.

On a perfectly sunny summer day, the time of year that you find hundreds of city dwellers and tourists sunbathing or throwing Frisbees at the Great Lawn in Central Park, I perform my small part on *All My Children*. My original plan was to lose eight pounds, so that I wouldn't look fat on television. I didn't lose the eight pounds, but I am having a "skinny" day, which makes all the difference in my attitude. I feel a little like a celebrity. There's an artist to do my hair and makeup, and people to assess my wardrobe. They give me "cookies" to put in my shirt to augment my flat chest.

The set is a Western motif, with a wooden bar and barstools, and peanut shells scattered around the floor. The actors drink out of beer mugs filled with colored water. The choreographer teaches us a country jig of a sort, with country line dancing and all. I stand in between Kelly Ripa and her on- and off-screen husband, Mark Consuelos.

Mark turns to me at one point and says, "Good thing you're standing there. I'm not much of a dancer. I'll just follow along with you."

Mark Consuelos talked to *moi*? I'm starstruck.

"Oh yeah, no problem. That's what we're here for," I responded, trying to act like I'm not talking to a celebrity. *That's what we're here for? You have one opportunity to speak to a celebrity and this is what you say? Can you say, dork?*

Of all the celebrities I encountered, Kelly Ripa leaves the largest impression. She is ridiculously skinny. I'd love to shove her into a room with Sarah Jessica Parker, a celeb with an equally childlike stature, for a cheeseburger-eating contest. The camera truly adds ten pounds, maybe more in her case.

Somehow the ultra skinny celebs seem to have a better grip on their lives than the anorexics I constantly see in Whole Foods, obsessing about which fantastic veggie burger mix to pair with their steamed haricots verts, or sitting on a lonely cafe corner taking an hour to suck down a twelve-ounce fat-free, dairy-free fruit smoothie. I really can't judge. I'm sure I, too, look odd to shoppers who see my tongue orally pleasuring the insides of the four or five Bavarian Cream donuts I'm eating, licking up every last bit of the yellow filling, while pushing my cart up and down the same three aisles of the grocery store deciding what to buy for dinner.

IN JULY, THANKS to my father who paid for my international flight, I fly with my dance teacher Michele and new roommates to the southern tip of Italy. Our trip is for three weeks, of which eight hours a day will be spent dancing on an Italian mountainside overlooking Sicily in the distance. A breathtaking landscape. I'm nervous thinking about eating pasta, pizza, and gelato. And I don't know what the bathroom situation will be like. I pack my suitcase with Balance Bars and Ziploc plastic bags full of my favorite almond-raisin combo to prevent any bingeing and purging. Typically, I can't eat almonds and raisins, as I regularly puke them up. But I decide it will be okay for this situation. I don't want to ruin my trip. Not only are we in Italy to be Michele's assistants, but we'll be assisting other well-known teachers too, including Terry Beeman, A.C. Ciulla, and Mia Michaels.

The first few days go extremely well. We dance. We sunbathe. We have wonderful conversations about dance and life. I feel like I'm a part of something. I feel, for once, that I am enough. I abstain from purging for three days.

Then everything changes.

On the fourth day, fifteen minutes into one of Michele's classes, I lean forward to stretch my back, a warm-up move I do everyday, and suddenly I feel my back tighten and spasm. My back is out. Laid up for a week, I choose to do nothing but lie in my villa and think about how depressing my life is and how I'm missing out and getting fat with this forced inactivity. After the first couple of days of rest, I can move around, but I'm still unable to dance, which makes me antsy. With my friends in class for eight hours, I start pacing around the white-tiled, white-walled villa. When I think of villa, I imagine the casita that sits above my extended family's house in Cabo San Lucas. This is no Italian villa. This is a room with four bare walls, two twin beds, and a bathroom.

Eventually, I begin plowing through my suitcase full of healthy snacks. I'm doing a dance of a sort: eat, purge, flush; eat, purge, flush. Eight hours a day. I keep this rhythm of destruction up for three days, until I go to flush the toilet on the third day and it doesn't flush. I've clogged the damn Italian toilet. Fuck. With only twenty minutes before class lets out, I dig my hands through the "healthy" mixture in the toilet. I scoop up handfuls of barely digested Balance Bars and transfer them from the pearly white toilet to a white plastic trash bag until I've scooped up just enough to unclog the toilet. Although I (thankfully) haven't had all that much practice at this, I accomplish the task before me at lightning speed.

Suddenly, with my arm still in the toilet, I hear Elizabeta's voice as she enters the villa.

"Oh, Hi, Elizabeta," I say, from behind the closed bathroom door, my heart now racing with adrenaline from the thought of being caught. "I'll be right out. I'm just going to the bathroom."

I flush the toilet and race over to the sink, quietly washing off the byproduct of my purge. The vestiges of my binge are up to my forearm, coating me like an intricately beaded tan glove. The grainy bits of nuts and nougat smooth my skin as I scrub them off, leaving my skin feeling unexpectedly silky. Who knew such an act of emesis could exfoliate the skin? *Hmm, almond, nutty, leaves the skin smooth and silky* . . . sounds like a perfect product to add to the shelves of Sephora. I could call it, *la purge de la peau*. No, maybe Italian inspired *il spurgo della pelle*. I'll have to think more about a name when I return to the States.

Once cleaned up, I look in the mirror and realize I've gotten away with it. *No one will ever know.*

Halfway through the trip, Michele, who notices something is off about me, wants to know the details. We take a walk down a little dirt road until we park ourselves at a secluded set of table and chairs to have a long conversation about my eating disorder. We've talked about it periodically in the past, but I've never given her the gory details of my struggles. She is the woman-of-the-hour I'm hoping will rescue me. She's uncharacteristically warm and sympathetic to my story, even a bit teary at times.

"You know, you're so talented. I care about you so much. You're worth so much more," Michele says to me.

"I just feel so, so empty. It never goes away."

"Just know that I love you, honey."

Sick equals love.

The only time my emptiness subsides is in class when I'm impressing my teachers. If they don't comment on my wonderful performance, I feel empty. If they don't give me constructive criticism, I feel empty. If they don't look at me, I feel empty. Even when they do all of these things, the fulfillment is somewhat fleeting. I feel high from the approval and attention briefly, but then I have to do more to sustain the high. I'm an approval and attention junkie, waiting for my next hit.

It isn't that I want Michele, or anyone else, to feel sorry for me. I just want someone who will validate my feelings and nurture me. God knows I can't do this for myself. I'm like an injured baby bird whose cut her wing, in constant search of the mama bird that will stop the bleeding and nurse my injury back to health. *Someone* has to take care of me.

"Have you tried Reiki?" she asks.

"No, it's too expensive." At $250 a pop, it exceeds my means.

"When we get back to the city, I'll take you to see my friend, Bill, who does Reiki. It releases all of the negative energy, and helps heal the soul." Yes, my soul needs healing. Michele must really care about me.

The remaining ten days of the trip go well, my back now feeling normal. I only purge the couple of times we go into town for pasta and gelato.

AFTER MY TRIP to Europe, I have to move. Once again, my eating has impeded on my ability to be an appropriate roommate. I find an apartment in Astoria Queens for $1,600 a month to share with my friend Marcy from Kansas City. She's moving to New York in a month. It's only a couple of stops from Manhattan, and it will be an easy commute to Radio City.

Marcy informs me that she will be toting her boyfriend Bobby along, which I'm not thrilled about. I don't like living with multiple people. Multiple roommates mean more people to notice my eating disorder. More people to confront me when we have house meetings. But, I am going to be busy. I probably won't be seeing them much anyway.

In early fall, rehearsals begin for the New York version of the *Radio City Christmas Spectacular*. And spectacular it is. We only have three weeks to put up the entire show—camels, little people, ice skaters and all—so we're rehearsing all day, practically every day.

On the first day, all thirty-six Rockettes, plus the "swings" and our dance captain, Sherry, sit in the Large Rehearsal Hall, listening to James L. Dolan, the CEO of Cablevision Systems, who oversees Madison Square Gardens and Radio City Entertainment. He expresses how excited he is to have all of us here. I'm amazed that

I'm included. *I don't belong in this room full of beauties.* Just like in Branson, most of the women have perfect, milky skin and luxurious long hair, which explains how, not just one, but several of them have grabbed pageant titles like Miss Louisiana or Miss Tennessee. I'm sure those in charge are questioning why they hired me.

Mr. Dolan tells us about the gifts we'll receive from our corporate sponsors, such as Capezio, bra reimbursements, gym membership discounts, discounted Madison Square Garden tickets, and the free cable that will begin three months after our hire date. He charms us further by mentioning The Rockette 401K plan, our year-round health insurance, and *Future Kicks*, a program that provides compensation for education to allow for a smooth transition from professional dancing to a new career. The perks are impressive.

After his speech, we go into the dressing room for our weigh-in. In addition, all Rockettes must undergo body composition tests, where a contracted company comes in and pinches our skin in various places, under our arms, on top of our thighs, on the side of our abdomen, to measure muscle and fat ratios. If a Rockette needs to lose weight, she will be warned. After two warnings, she may be suspended without pay. When a Rockette corrects her actions, she will be notified in writing by management that she has been taken off warning. After three, she may be dismissed.

While I know this is just part of the job—similar to knowing that taking up a career in data entry could lead to carpal tunnel syndrome—the external focus on aesthetic ideals is exactly the type of societal nemesis that fuels the neuroses of young girls and women to be hypervigilant about their appearance.

Performing in Branson, I never had any problems with weight. The gay boys in the show loved my body, saying that I had the best legs of the bunch. Even Trina, the assistant choreographer who has amazing legs herself, commented on how beautiful my legs were.

There were girls during both my first and second season, however, who were called into the office and given a warning to shape up, literally. I knew I needed to stay thin to avoid that kind of humiliation.

Now though, as I've put on at least ten pounds since my Branson days, I'm a little nervous.

"I know that no one wants to get weighed, but we have to do it. It's no big deal. I'm sure most of you have nothing to worry about," the assistant says.

When it's my turn, I tiptoe onto the scale, hoping it won't register the entire weight of me.

"136 and a half," the assistant reads aloud.

Ouch. *See, if you would've just followed your food plan, you would be skinny by now.* I want to weigh less, much less. She writes my weight down in a spiral notebook and says nothing more.

I AM ON the heavier side, compared to many of the other women, some who run five miles to work before performing four shows in a day. But I'm not the heaviest, thank God.

"If we feel you need to lose weight, you'll be notified in writing."

That's that. *I'd better lose weight,* I admonish myself, *just in case I'm on the fat list.*

After the weigh-in, we break for lunch. I've brought a turkey sandwich and a peach. There is no way I'm going to binge and purge. Immediately after, we have media training, which is where each of us has to stand before a camera, performing a mock interview, to see who can gracefully spit out lines like, "The *Radio City Christmas Spectacular* provides fun for the whole family!" on cue for the gamut of publicity events that occur during the holiday season. I absolutely loathe this exercise. I already know that I can't speak well in front of a camera, as I've had to do this publicity practice twice before in Branson.

They ask us random questions that a reporter or interviewer

would ask to see how quickly we respond with the correct answer. We're instructed to never say "The Show" or "The Rockettes," when speaking of The *Radio City Christmas Spectacular* starring the Radio City Rockettes. It's a mouthful, but one I'm proud to say correctly.

Trying to maintain a positive perspective, I've decided that when my name is called this year, I'll be ready. I'm not going to let my nerves get the best of me. *Greta, you're an excellent public speaker.* Silently, I practice responding to the range of random questions they might ask in their effort to see how quickly and eloquently I can respond. *It's mind over matter, that's all. There isn't anything these other girls have over you.* I don't really buy the bullshit I'm feeding my brain, but I repeat my confidence boosters until I'm summoned.

"So tell me, why do you love dancing as a Radio City Rockette?" the mock interviewer asks me. I can feel the room watching me.

I stand there smiling, saying nothing for what feels like three minutes, trying not to worry about the bright spotlight of the camera highlighting my acne scars. *Excuse me, what was the question? Why do I love being a Rockette? Being a Rockette . . . what did she ask me?*

I finally remember the question, gather myself, and begin pondering what I actually do love about dancing as a Radio City Rockette. There are many things I love . . . the organization, the costumes, dancing at the Music Hall . . . the money . . . but, of course, that isn't the correct answer. I had drawn a blank.

The interviewer probes me with a supportive, but hurrying smile.

"I love being a Rockette because the *Radio City Christmas Spectacular* is fun for the whole family!" I had answered a question, but not the one she'd asked me. And I'd said "Rockette" instead of "Radio City Rockette." After other girls had done their interviews, there had been whispers about how great she did. After mine, there is just a lifeless courtesy applause. There's nothing, really, to comment on. I had totally sucked. *No, I won't be doing any interviews this year.*

My face is hot with shame and embarrassment. I can never be normal. I feel like I don't ever fully fit in. I can't fully relax, especially when all of those women are staring at and judging me. I feel like the oddball of the bunch who barely made it.

"Who's up next?" the assistant asks, moving on from my wayward mock interview.

REHEARSALS ARE LONG, but fruitful. In the Large Rehearsal Hall, toward the front of the studio, by the wall of mirrors, there's a long number line taped to the floor. Every transition in the choreography is based on the number line. It is our guide to keep us in check about where we should be at all times. In some routines, we move as many as twenty different times, so skillful memorization is imperative.

Often during rehearsals, Mark or Lynn will stand directly in front of me, or any one of us, study the line with a serious squint, and say, "Greta, can you move over one quarter of an inch?" *One quarter of an inch.* The perfection required is incredible. It has to be. Precision dance and kicks are what make the Radio City Rockettes a world-famous organization.

We take in a massive amount of information, which the director expects us to perfectly retain when he calls out the names of the routines to rehearse, now reduced to informal abbreviations like "Ragdolls," "Reindeers," and "Wreaths." After the first two weeks of rehearsal, we transition from the Large Rehearsal Hall to the stage.

Radio City Music Hall describes it best: "The Great Stage, as it's called, because of legendary entertainers who've performed there, from Frank Sinatra to Martha Graham to Madonna, truly is an absolutely amazing place to perform. Because there are no columns to obstruct views, virtually every seat is a superb seat, which is one of the many reasons why the Great Stage is considered by technical experts to be the most perfectly equipped anywhere."

Besides setting the show on the stage, we do costume run-throughs to practice the many Rockette thirty-second quick-changes. Our costumes are preset in various places, on the sides of stage right and stage left, with dressers close by, waiting to zip, snap, and buckle. In numbers like "Santa Claus" and "Reindeers," we surprise the audience by entering from below stage level. We rise on a rotating platform; so, we have our brown velvet reindeer unitard, antler headpiece, tap shoes, and Santa suits set below.

On opening night, as I step foot onto the stage, smiling through the bushy green wreath that frames my face, I know what the veterans mean when they say there is nothing like stepping onto that stage. I can't see many faces in the audience because of the bright spotlight honing in on our line of thirty-six; but I can hear the screams of the six thousand people cheering for us. *It is awesome.*

We barrel through the show, performing "Need a Little Christmas," "The Parade of the Wooden Soldiers," and "Christmas in New York" in the first act; and "Mannequins," "Ragdolls," "Santas," "Reindeers," and "Nativity" in the second act. Besides the usual opening night kinks, like a dropped prop or incorrect timing on a set change, the show goes smoothly. I'm in the "big leagues" and it feels marvelous!

The following day, I receive a call from my mother.

"Hi, Greta. So, how did the shows go?"

"Everything went smoothly. No major mistakes."

"Did it feel cool to dance on that stage with all of the people?" The excited tone of her voice lets me know that my mother is really proud of me.

"Yes, it was awesome."

"How are the other dancers? Do you like them?"

"Oh, yeah. Everyone's pretty cool." I had made some friends. Becky, who I danced with in Branson, had become one of my close friends. And Heather, who sat next to me in the dressing room, was really friendly. I wasn't about to mention the slew of bitchy women who treated me as if I was a communicable disease.

"Well, Grandma Patty, Pam, Sherry, and I have our New York City trip planned."

"Great! When are you coming?" I can't wait for my family to visit.

"Sometime in late November. And, of course, we will have to go to the *Today Show*. We'll have to figure out a gimmick so that we get on television. And we will have to do the double-decker bus tour."

"Yeah, definitely," I say. "I'm sure you guys will figure out something to get on television. You all are so creative."

"Uh-huh . . . so . . . how's the weather? I saw on the *Today Show* that it looks pretty nice." My mood takes on an almost Pavlovian shift when I hear the word weather. When there is nothing more to say, we revert to safe weather talk, which annoys the fuck out of me.

"It's fine. Not too cold yet." There's a long silence. I'm waiting for my mom to say something. "Hello?" I say to see if she's still on the other end.

"Yeah, I'm here. Well, I guess that's about all," she says. I'm enraged at this point. *How can that be all? Nothing more to say? How about my eating disorder? There's a topic. Why don't you ever tell me how much you care, or how valuable I am as a human being, or how I don't need to harm myself? Give me something.*

There has to be more to our relationship than this. I wonder if, in between the spaces of our empty dialogue, she feels it, too. Is she aware of our conversations' lackluster content? Of course, I don't mention any of my feelings either. I resentfully participate in our empty conversations, swallowing my anger with every word.

"Well, I guess I'll talk to you later," I say.

"Okay. Have a good week."

"You too," I say. I throw the phone down on my bed. I want to scream. I don't know how to deal with any emotions that are uncomfortable. Anger, anxiety, fear, sadness, loss—I do anything to push these feelings down. It is only acceptable to feel happiness. I have to get out of here. I grab my backpack and a pack of Marlboro Lights.

I started smoking years ago when I was on a dance scholarship in Los Angeles. I barely was able to inhale. A lot of the dancers smoked. So cliché. Now, I smoke a pack a day. It's my only other coping mechanism besides throwing up. Sometimes, smoking even helps distract me from being hungry. Other times, it helps me not to purge after a meal because it squashes my anxiety about feeling full. It's just one other crutch in my life.

I come out of my bedroom to see my roommate, Marcy, in the kitchen eating breakfast.

"Hey, what's up?" she asks. I rarely see or talk to Marcy anymore. She and her boyfriend mostly hide out in their room or go out to clubs. I mostly binge and purge in my room. It doesn't leave a lot of time for small talk.

"Hey," I say. "I'm going out. Be back in a bit."

"Okay. I probably won't see you. I have to work."

"Is Bobby working, too?"

"Yeah, he's one of the closers at the restaurant tonight."

"Oh, okay. Then I guess I'll see you when I see you." Knowing they will both be out of the house sends excitement through my body. I can binge and purge all night.

I leave my apartment and escape to one of the many Greek diners in Astoria. I come here often to drown my anger in syrupy pancakes and French fries with mayonnaise.

SINCE OUR OPENING performance, the director, choreographer, and assistants sit in the audience to take notes for each routine.

These are the miniscule details that the audience never notice, but are important to ensure the precision required to fulfill our job description. If one of the routines needs a lot of work, then we have to schedule additional rehearsal time in between shows. If we really suck, rehearsals can occur several times a week. Just what I love to do is spend my break rehearsing someone else's screw up, free of charge!

One of the most infamous numbers in the show is "The Parade of the Wooden Soldiers." After the opening "Wreath" number, we scurry into the elevator and ride up to our dressing room on the fifth floor to put on our soldier costume. I quickly unpeel my tan sparkle tights from my now warmed-up legs, and change from my silver t-strap tap shoes into my black t-strap taps. I tape cutout red circles to my real cheeks, and put on ultra starched white pants and a red and blue soldier jacket.

Our pants have to be extra stiff so that it doesn't look like we're walking with bent knees onstage, which would take away the wooden-soldier effect. When starched just enough, our pants can stand up on their own. Sometimes we put a few pairs of pants in a line and take a picture. It's actually pretty comical, in the spirit of David Byrne's big white suit from *Stop Making Sense*.

The last piece of our costume is the black soldier hat. To ensure that the hat is aligned correctly, making each dancer's hat stand at the precise vertical angle, we put our hats on and stand with our backs against a wall. Once the brim of the hat lowers to meet our eyes, with just enough eyeshot of light that we can see the number line onstage, we know it's perfect. The hat strap has to tighten as much as possible without strangling our necks, so it doesn't bob back and forth. Once again, I realize it's the precision and detail that makes our shows what they are.

Performed since 1933, "Parade" is a crowd-pleaser because the children believe that we are real-life toy soldiers, and the adults are in awe of our perfect pinwheels and line formations. Merely walking like a wooden soldier is a tiresome task. Out of the stage gate, with our arms glued to our sides, we lift our hip ever so slightly with each step we take, giving us a completely straight-legged walk. Not to mention, it's a great hip trimmer! Occasionally, I will turn my head sharply the wrong way during the performance, to find all of the other Rockettes looking in my direction. The girl next to me will giggle through her glued-shut lips, as I shout a ventriloquist's, "Oh, Fuck!" When this happens, the trick is to figure out how to turn my head the correct way without the audience noticing. More importantly, I don't want our choreographer, who's taking notes in the audience, to see my slip up.

The highlight of the "Parade of the Wooden Soldiers" is the great soldier fall. After having danced uniform for the whole routine, something goes haywire, and we, the wooden soldiers, begin to go crazy, moving sporadically, then fitfully, around the stage. After we somehow find our way to a straight line, we sharply turn to the side, showing the audience our profiles, and shoot our hands stiffly onto the hips of the soldier in front of us. The big boom of a canon ball signals the beginning of the great soldier fall.

Beginning with the first soldier on stage left, the soldier fall has a very specific technique. Each soldier does the same four moves, timed by watching the soldier in front of you, as well as the momentum of the fall. Because the first soldier on stage left doesn't have anyone in front of her, she simply leans back at the appropriate time. The second soldier in line takes her hands that are on the first soldier's hips and slides them up to her armpits. From there, she pulls the soldier backwards, in a very controlled manner, into her chest, while simultaneously shooting her hands through her armpits, making two fists, bringing them upward and in, so they're hugging her chest. Then, the second soldier lifts her elbows out to the side to lock the first soldier in place. While this is happening, the second soldier also lifts her toes off the ground, so that she is now balancing on the heels of her tap shoes, ready to fall backwards. This technique continues down the line, gradually picking up speed.

While the fall captivates the audience, if done incorrectly this well-orchestrated and much-rehearsed maneuver can be quite dangerous. The most important part of the soldier fall is to keep your knees locked straight and your abdominal muscles tight, especially when you fall backwards. If a soldier relaxes her body, then she isn't going to be able to control the weight from the soldiers in front of her. This will send the line slamming backwards, forcing anonymous grunts and quiet yelps to shoot from our mouths, as the girl's chest in front barrels into the soldier behind her. The soldiers in the back of the line become vulnerable to knee or back injuries. All of the Rockettes get pissed if a girl doesn't pull her weight. And if it goes badly during a performance, the choreographer and dance captain make us rehearse the soldier fall in between shows, which no one likes.

While I concentrated so hard on my own technique each show, making it my goal to never receive a note from the choreographer in the audience, I could feel that I was entering the beginning of my own great fall. I knew that a day would come where I'd bend my knees, relax my body, feel the weight of my decisions slam into me . . . and just let everything go.

Even with three or four shows a day, I can't control my eating. Every week when I receive my paycheck, I vow to not spend it all on binge food, yet by the end of the week, I'm practically out of money. I confide in my friend, Heather, a Rockette whose assigned spot in the dressing room is next to mine. She gives me a quick solution: follow a low glycemic diet, which will provide me with five to six small meals a day, so I won't ever be hungry. She also gives me her recipe for egg white and oatmeal pancakes and a workout regimen. I review my library of books on anorexia, trying to get thinspiration so that I can control myself. Nothing works. I can't stop bingeing and purging.

Even though I was never one of the Rockettes told to lose weight, at 137 pounds I'm tipping the scales, almost entering the devastating categories of chunky and untoned. To add to the matter, the New York show is much less physically demanding and doesn't burn as many calories as I'd expected based on previous experiences in the CONY shows. Between the thick velvet green outfits that we wear for the opening number and the two layers of tights, one pair of Capezio tan tights and a thicker sparkle Lycra tight, I feel like I'm busting at every seam.

I'm living a dual life. Everyday, I take the N train from Astoria, carting myself to the Music Hall, take the elevator up to the fifth floor to my dressing room, and greet my friends with a smile on my face. I sit in the dressing room in my tan show bra and tan tights, laughing and stretching with the other girls, while I get ready for the opening act.

What they don't know is that while I'm sitting at my dressing table putting on my fake eyelashes and sparkly earrings, I'm berating myself intensely. As I look at my acne-scarred face, I'm thinking about how pretty all of the other girls are, compared to myself, and I'm scrutinizing the folds of skin on my stomach, disgusted by the fat rolls. I look at Mia's spunky personality and wish I could be that free. So many of the women have six-pack abs. I used to, when I was really thin. All of the girls have clear skin; many have doe-shaped eyes. Listening to Tina sing in the dressing room, I realize I probably will never perform on Broadway because I can't sing. Precision dance may be the only job I'm cut out for. Most of all, these women are confident. At least they appear to be. They aren't needy emotional sponges. I doubt they are having the negative self-talk I'm having now.

I'm not thinking about the notes given to me by our dance captain after the previous show that I need to employ today. My mind is not anywhere close to being on the show. I'm in planning and calculation mode. Planning my food and calculating calories. I'm planning my binges, too, calculating the amount of time I can binge and purge until I have to be back for another show, or how many hours I will be alone to eat in solace at my apartment.

The other Rockettes don't realize that while they carry on, chattering about what song they will sing at their next audition or changing their hair color from platinum blond to brunette, because it may increase their marketability, I'm thinking about if and how I should kill myself. *A bottle of benzodiazepines or two vertical slices to the wrists? Who will I write notes to?* I entertain myself with suicidal ideation at least every other day. They don't realize that on our long break during shows, instead of resting I'm gorging myself at the Dean & Deluca gourmet deli in the Rockefeller Complex.

I lead a spectacular life.

Interlude

I was five years old the first time I realized I loved food. The details around the event are somewhat muddled, but I do know that it was a Friday, because on Fridays my preschool teacher made our class special snacks. There I sat, on the carpet of my Catholic preschool in prayer stance, but I wasn't praying. I was watching the constant whip, whip, whip of the rubber spatula that Mrs. Blackburn used to churn the homemade butter that would accompany the saltine crackers we were having for snack. Entranced, I sat wide-eyed with fascination, and my mouth watered as I imagined the heavenly cream fluff caressing my palate.

Our allotment was three crackers with butter; however, I needed more. I didn't know why, I just knew that I needed more. I relished in the comfort that seeped into my taste buds, bite after bite, spreading a tarp of security across my tongue. As I neared the end of my third cracker, I silently yearned for more. Clouds of shame and embarrassment cast their shadows over me, diluting my desires. I knew that I wasn't supposed to want more.

No one told me I shouldn't want more. Intrinsically, I just knew.

I knew right then that I had a different relationship with food than my classmates. They weren't disappointed that they had finished their crackers. Pleasure didn't envelop every orifice of their bodies when imagining stuffing as many butter-and-cracker duos down their throats as they could shovel in. No, they didn't have a relationship with food; they didn't even think about food; they just ate when they were hungry and stopped when they were full. What a concept. As I sulked silently in the corner of my Catholic preschool that day, I didn't realize that in that instant, the god I was praying to, the god I was looking toward for solace and serenity was food.

I knew my relationship with food was somewhat peculiar, but I didn't realize the full extent of our relationship until I was eight years old. Many afternoons after school, I'd go over to Colleen Hall's house. Colleen and I had been best friends since the first grade. We were inseparable, thoroughly delighted to spend our afternoons playing school or office together, acting as if we were teachers or CEOs of a big corporation. On our pretend lunch break, Colleen and I frequently paced her kitchen floor and rummaged through her kitchen cabinets in search of the perfect snack to nibble on.

One day, when we were in Colleen's kitchen eating a snack, something clicked in my brain and I have never been the same since.

Colleen grabs a bag of chips from the cabinet.

"Hey, let's act like we're the Cookie Monster and shove chips into our mouths," Colleen says.

"Okay," I reply. It sounds fun to me.

I stick my hand deep into the bag of potato chips, grab the largest handful of potato chips I can, and shove my hand into my mouth. Greasy remnants of chips scatter themselves across my face, but I don't care. I continue to shove chips into my mouth, this time two-handedly. With each salty swallow, layers of comfort coat my throat as the food slides down, creating a fullness of pleasure throughout my body. An overwhelming sense of calmness showers me. My skin stops crawling. I'm no longer nervous. Almost as quickly as the feeling washes over me, it dissipates. *I want that feeling back.*

It is here, standing in the kitchen at eight years old, that I make a subconscious pact with food. *I've found my lover. We will be together forever.*

My fondest memories of food, as well as childhood, are at my grandmother's house. Starting at the age of six, Grandma Sally picks me up from school on Fridays. With bright pink lipstick and her teased perm, which she has washed every Wednesday at the Jones Store beauty salon, my grandmother always looks ready to hit the bowling alley with "her gals." She always smells like a bottle of Estée Lauder's White Linen perfume. Nicknamed "Sally Bags," because she sells handbags at the Jones Store Company, Grandma Sally is very religious, attending Catholic mass regularly.

Like a good Catholic, she never hesitates before shouting profanities at the television whenever the Kansas City Royals are losing. With exception to her filthy mouth, she is the epitome of a saint, or at least the psychological equivalent of a codependent, always bending over backward for everyone else and putting herself last. Because I'm an only child and the first grandchild, Grandma Sally and I have a very special relationship. She calls me "Greta the Great." I can do no wrong in her eyes.

Every Friday, on the way to my grandparents' house, Grandma Sally and I drive to the Village, a small shopping mall near her house, where we stop at Bruce Smith's drugstore for some sweet treats. Grandma is a long-standing customer, forty years at least, so all of the employees know her. Bells jingle above our heads as we walk through the glass front door. Grandma waves to one of the cashiers, Betty, across the store.

"Greta," Grandma Sally says. "I'm going to pick up Gramps'

medicine and talk to Betty for a minute." Gramps takes heart pills and shots for diabetes. "Why don't you go and pick out your candy."

I race over to the candy aisle. There are so many choices— nuts, marshmallows, peanut butter, milk chocolate. I stare at the three-tiered rack of candy in front of me and deliberate carefully, trying to decide which bar, nut, or nougat will fulfill me the most. It's a tough call. Reese's? M&M's? Milky Way? Kit Kat? My eyes scan the candy selections repeatedly, the way my Jackson 5 record repeats itself when it skips. I go through this methodical ritual every Friday. From the second shelf, I grab a Hershey's bar and a Reese's Peanut Butter Cup. Just having the chocolate in my hand boosts my security level. I can barely resist opening the candy before we arrive at Grandma's.

I'm not sure why, but she says the same thing every time I walk through the front door of my grandparents' itty-bitty two-bedroom house.

"Oh, this house is filthy! Don't look at the dust."

I don't care. I love it. It's much different from my house, where every antique rug or Asian artifact has a place, and every morsel of food is monitored. My parents are obsessed with dieting. They do keep some junk food in the house, but my parents notice every chip, cracker, or cookie consumed.

When Daddy comes home from work, he walks directly to the kitchen cabinets to grab a snack. He first eats a few Triscuits, followed by a few handfuls of Ruffles potato chips.

He shakes the bag. "Who ate my Ruffles? Greta, did you eat my potato chips?"

"I only ate a few," I lie.

"I don't think so. Yesterday there was half a bag left."

"I told you, Daddy, I only ate a little bit." I always stick to my story.

My father's a yo-yo dieter who vacillates between food restriction and overeating, dropping and gaining ten or twenty pounds at a time. He's obsessed with the scale. Even on "good" weigh-in days, he isn't satisfied.

"Yeah, I lost ten pounds. I feel better," he will say. "But in five or ten more pounds, I should be in pretty good shape."

Losing any amount of weight gives my father the green light to overeat at dinner. Every night, he sprints through his dinner, using his fork to hurdle over the mounds of mashed potatoes and meat piled high on his plate. He stuffs himself to the brim, and then lets out a long, loud burp, so that he can shove in the final bites of his dinner and cross over the clean-plate-club finish line.

"Ugh. I shouldn't have eaten that much. I feel sick." His closing remark is always the same.

My dad also likes to manage my mother's weight.

"Okay, Gayle," Daddy demands on some mornings. "Let's see your weight."

She steps cautiously onto the scale. 126. She exhales a sigh of relief as she reads the number on the digital scale.

"Jeez-us!" my dad sarcastically exclaims. "Look at your weight! Must be that big ass." My father was cruel about her appearance. After many meals, my mom would wrap her arm around her waist and feel her side, where a love handle would be if she actually had one.

"What are you doing?" I'd say, watching her pinch her side.

"Checking to see how fat I am."

My mother is just as neurotic about her food intake as she is about everyone else's. She has a set of food rules for herself that she tries to transfer onto my father and me. Rules about what my father and I are allowed to have.

"Greta," she will say, as she watches me take four or five Oreo cookies. "You only need to take two. You don't want to get fat now, do you?"

She has other rules, too, rules that aren't necessarily spoken. My mother's ideology shoots through in a single look. A look that says, *You aren't going to eat another bite are you? I can't believe you're going to keep going. You've had enough.*

Like a hawk, she examines every spread of mayonnaise and dollop of butter that accompanies my plate. I hate her looks. I know that her eye of judgment stems from fear that originates and resides in her, but somehow transfers to me across our enmeshed boundaries. The fear of: "If you eat another bite, you might get fat; and if you're fat, then no one will like you, you won't look good in clothes, and you will never be able to get a boyfriend or a husband, the person who will someday take care of you." Yes, for my mother it has always been about the end goal—the boyfriend.

How unfortunate it will be for her when I tell her that I'm a lesbian.

Grandma Sally doesn't share any of my parents' philosophies. She encourages me to eat. In fact, she is concerned that I don't have enough food to eat.

"Honey, can I fix you something? A pizza? A sandwich? I don't want you to starve."

At my grandparents' house, starving is impossible. Every Friday is the same. I begin my four-course meal with the candy I picked out from the drugstore. I'm a food chemist. I alternate between bites of chocolate and Diet Pepsi to create the perfect chemical compound to boost my naturally low serotonin level and elevate my psyche to a plateau of pleasure. I savor every bite, wishing it could last forever.

My food frenzy continues as I walk into her kitchen across the cream linoleum and take a sleeve of saltine crackers from the tin container. I take the Kraft Deluxe American cheese out of the fridge and pull out three or four slices. My fingertips glide across the smooth creamy surface. Soft as silk. I fold each slice into perfect quarters and layer them in between my saltines until I have built a tower of comfort. I balance the tower in the palm of my hand, as though I'm performing a trick, as I walk back into the living room. I sink into the couch and proceed to eat them, one by one.

"Greta," Grandma calls from the kitchen. "Be sure to save room for dinner. I don't want you to get a tummy ache."

"Don't worry, Grandma. I won't."

As I finish my last cracker, an emotional lull hits me. I don't know what to do with myself now. My eyes bounce from the television to the clock, back to the television, once again to the clock, the television, the clock, back and forth, for the next forty-five minutes. I try to be engrossed in *The Brady Bunch* to keep myself from obsessing about the macaroni and cheese dinner that's baking and bubbling in the oven.

Every Friday at 6:30 PM, my mother promptly arrives from work to my grandparents' house to eat dinner with us. While Grandma Sally finishes preparing dinner, my mother and I sit in the kitchen. Every Friday, we exchange audio clips of empty chatter to help pass the time.

My mother always begins. "How was your day, Greta?"

I start telling her about my day at school, but I can tell by her uh-huhs that, rather than listening to me, she is examining me. Her eyes scan my body from head to toe. I feel exposed but carry on as if I don't notice. Her eyes stop at my abdomen.

"Greta, stick in your stomach."

I was eight years old the first time I heard those words, stick in your stomach. Both at home as well as in dance class. More than the words, it was the look I remember. Like, *how ridiculous that you would stick out your stomach.* Looking back, I'm sure that my mom meant it as a casual comment, with no malicious intent. But, for whatever reason, I clung to words and looks from my mother and other authority figures, allowing them to influence my emotions and how I felt about myself as a human being.

From those four words—stick in your stomach—emerged a belief system about myself. At this tender age of eight, I became acutely aware that how I externally appeared mattered in some way. From that day forward, I attempted to keep my stomach sucked in at all times, whether in public or in the privacy of my own room playing with Barbie dolls.

"Dinner's ready!" yells Grandma Sally, her signal to Gramps to turn his hearing aids back on and join us in the dining room.

I spoon a healthy portion of macaroni and cheese onto my plate. I need more. I want to devour the luscious plate of macaroni and cheese sitting in front of me, but instead take careful bites to savor every moment. Layered with butter, flour, and Kraft Deluxe American cheese, my grandmother's macaroni and cheese is my favorite meal. Nestled within each layer lies a depth and fullness that I desperately need. It's my crack cocaine. If I could inject it into my veins, I would. With each bite, the creamy consistency effortlessly glides down my throat, attaching itself to every spore of emptiness encompassing my body before inching its way down to my stomach. Before I've even finished my first helping, my mind fantasizes about the next.

After dinner, I volunteer to put our plates away so that I can sneak in a couple slivers of the Sara Lee coffee cake we're having for dessert. I'm stuffed from dinner, but I don't care. All I want now is that buttery sweet coffee cake.

The Great Fall of One Wooden Soldier

In late November, I cart myself off to the morning Overeaters Anonymous meeting on the Upper West Side. My role as a Rockette has not cured my eating disorder, and it hasn't provided me with the sense of self-love and confidence I had expected it would. It has, however, provided a consistent chunk of money every week, so the amount of time I spend bingeing and purging has increased. I am exhausted all of the time.

I walk into the church on Eighty-Sixth Street. The room is crowded. The 9:30 AM meeting is very popular. I take a seat in the circle of chairs. I see a few familiar faces. I really don't want to share that I'm relapsing. I like to appear as if I have it all together. As I hear people share about their gratitude for being abstinent or feeling hopeless about their most recent relapses, I keep eyeing the clock, trying to decide if I'm going to share my truth with the group. It's a toss up.

". . . So, for today, I'm not going to buy jeans, because I don't want to beat myself up about gaining the weight," says Shari, a middle-aged bulimic. "I'm going to . . . ."

"Time," a young woman says with her hand held out in a fist.

She's what we refer to in Overeaters Anonymous as the spiritual time-keeper. In about three seconds, I know I have to decide whether I'm going to raise my hand. *Three . . . two . . . one.*

"Thank you," Shari says. "I'm going to pray to my higher power to release me from my obsession with body image."

"Thank you, Shari," the room shouts.

My hand shoots up in the air, catching the timekeeper's attention. She chooses me.

"Hi, my name is Greta, and I'm a bulimic."

"Hi, Greta," the room shouts back.

"Well, my eating is just really bad right now," I begin. My eating hasn't ever been good, meaning without relapse, but I feel less shame if I present myself as if at one time I was in recovery. "I keep bingeing and purging. I'm in total relapse. I'm doing a dance job and making great money, which could be enough for me to save a lot of money. But because I'm spending so much on food, I'm practically living paycheck to paycheck. My life is so unmanageable. I just feel hopeless."

I don't actually believe that I will get better from coming to meetings. I've been coming to meetings for a long time now without ever achieving solid abstinence. The spiritual timekeeper holds her hand out, her index finger in the air. This is my one-minute warning.

"Anyway, I really need a sponsor. I'm just putting it out there. Thanks for letting me share."

"Thanks, Greta." I feel like a freak. Even though this is what food addicts talk about, I feel like I'm not supposed to be talking about my relapse. Others can, but not me. My ego has a lot of pride and doesn't want anyone to know that I'm fucking up. I hate to admit it, but it's true.

After the meeting, I do what I usually do: I go up to people to let them know that I took their phone number from the *We Care* book that was passed around at the meeting. I ask them if I can call them. "Anytime. Please call me," they will say. I have found that "anytime" doesn't really exist in the city. People have so much going on that I'm lucky if someone calls me back in the same day.

I make my way through the circle of chairs and clusters of duos and trios standing together, trying to reach my friend Katherine. She is talking to someone I don't know, which is always awkward for me. I'm standing off to the side from Katherine feeling like I'm eavesdropping on a conversation, but really I just want to say hello. Katherine sees me out of the corner of her eye.

"Hi, Katherine," I say, giving her a big hug. Katherine and I have known each other for several months now. She is a performer, too. She's a singer and dancer, and we sometimes take Michele's class together. But her heart lies in comedy writing. She takes classes at the Upright Citizen's Brigade.

"Hi, Greta. I'm so sorry you are struggling so much. Are you seeing a therapist?"

"No, I don't know of one. Plus, I'm not sure if I can afford to go."

"Well, I have an amazing therapist. She will probably work out a sliding scale with you."

"Really? What's her name?" Katherine digs in her Marc Jacobs bag. She pulls out a business card and hands it to me: Heather Karaman, CSW. I've always had the goal to someday be a clinical social worker. I've always wanted to help people with eating disorders. I just have to help myself first.

"Thanks, Katherine," I say, putting the card in my wallet for safekeeping.

After the meeting, I pull the card back out of my wallet and study it. Heather Karaman, CSW. She sounds nice on paper. If Katherine says she's great, then she probably is. I call the number on the card and leave a message.

The following Wednesday evening, I go to her office at Ninety-First Street between Park Avenue and Lexington. Heather buzzes me in.

"Hi, I'm Heather Karaman. It's lovely to meet you," she says. Heather is much younger than I imagined. She has long brown hair the color of dark chocolate, and big brown eyes. She's thin, not too thin, but thin enough. Her voice is distinct. She could be a former actress.

"You can have a seat," she says. The office epitomizes a NYC therapist's office. An inviting, quaint space, with a leather couch, stacks of books, exposed brick walls, and soft lighting.

I sit down on the patient couch. Heather stares at me for a moment.

"Greta, would you like to tell me what brought you here today?" This part—telling a stranger about the most secret parts of your life—is always a little awkward.

"Well . . . as I mentioned on the phone, I have an eating disorder." And so it begins. The shameful divulgence. "I'm a dancer. I dance as a Rockette at Radio City." I hope to impress her with my abilities and vocation, though I immediately feel embarrassed for having the need to want to impress her. *Attention-seeking asshole.* In a split second I go from feeling proud to feeling sure she's wondering how someone like me, with a big nose and acne-pitted cheeks, could possibly be a Rockette."

"A Rockette? How long have you been doing that for?"

"Yes. Well, this is my first year doing the New York show. I performed outside of New York for the last two years."

"I see. How long have you been struggling with bulimia?"

"Since I was sixteen years old," I say. Sixteen. I had no idea then that I'd still be in a full-blown eating disorder thirteen years later.

"You've struggled a long time," she says. As Heather takes me through her line of questions about my family, my work history, my upbringing, significant events—a standard psychosocial history—I can already feel the pull. I don't want to, but I feel it. The familiar emotional tug triggered by my sense of someone's genuine empathy for me.

"How many times a day are you purging?"

"Ten to twenty, give or take. I can't stand the feeling of fullness. When I binge, I eat a small amount and then purge every fifteen minutes or so. And then if I feel full when I try to eat on my food plan, I also have to purge."

"So feeling full is a major trigger?"

"Yes."

"You've had such a difficult time. How are your moods? Do you have a history of depression?"

"Yes. I went to a psychiatrist in Kansas, where I'm from, and he said I had dysthymia."

"Uh-huh. A type of low-grade depression that is always lying beneath the surface."

"Yes, exactly."

"When did that start?"

"After my parents divorce. Well, actually, I first started feeling depressed around eighth grade, which was before my eating disorder."

"What was going on then?"

"Some of it was typical teenage stuff. I was having problems with my friends. I felt uglier than all of them. I found out that my favorite ballet teacher would be leaving. My parents were always fighting. Something just sparked, and I had a sudden awareness of a level of unhappiness within me. It was as if I woke up to some bitter reality. I felt like everyone at school walked around carefree and laughing all of the time. I wondered what made them feel that happy. It was the first time, I guess, that I really hated myself."

"What was making you feel so ugly at the time?" *Isn't it obvious?*

"Well, I've always hated my nose. I broke it as a kid doing a front flip off the balance beam when I was in gymnastics. And then I had acne. It was something both my mom and dad always commented about. My mom would take a really hot washcloth and scrub the t-zone areas until they were red and practically raw. I think she tried to literally rub the acne right off my face. And then if I didn't wear foundation in public to cover up my acne, she would scream at me, wondering why I didn't care enough to make myself look good."

"That's a heartbreaking image, Greta."

"Well, I can deal with it now. During my first hospitalization—I've been hospitalized twice for my eating disorder—I couldn't talk about it without breaking down. But I've gotten used to it."

"And how about your father? You said he talked about it, too?"

"Yes, he would point and ask me how my acne was doing, whatever that means. But, it was more in a joking kind of a way. It's hard to describe, but he'd kind of point at my face like he was connecting my dots of acne. It wasn't malicious. My mom wasn't trying to be malicious either. She just wanted me to look the best that I could so that I'd have friends and be popular, and maybe get a boyfriend."

"That kind of joking doesn't sound too funny."

"I guess not. That's just him. He doesn't mean it in a bad way."

"You were hospitalized twice you said?"

"Yes. Both times for bulimia. The second time I was more of an anorexic weight—about twenty-five pounds lighter than I am now—but still purging at least a dozen times a day."

"Just from what you've told me so far, it sounds like you've had a lot going on."

"Yeah, I guess."

"Well, Greta, we only have a few minutes left. Does this time work for you?" Panic settles in. I hate when time is up. I never have enough time. Ever.

"Sure."

"Okay, so I'll see you next Wednesday at 6:30 PM. Have a good week, Greta," she says, standing up and motioning me toward the door.

"Can I give you a hug? I mean do we do that here?" My other therapists all hugged me after the first session.

"Yes, we can hug. I always wait until the patient initiates. I would never invade someone's boundaries."

Heather gives me a warm embrace, and then I make my exit.

Walking down Madison Avenue toward the Eighty-Sixth Street subway, I know Heather is already cast as my new savior who will take care of all emotional needs. The one whom I will not try to get better for; but, rather sicker for to gain and, more importantly, keep her love, care, and affection.

Sick equals love.

Five days later, my mom, Aunt Sherry, Aunt Pam, and Grandma Patty arrive to see me in the show. It's bad hair timing. My hair has been very short and it's in a weird growing out phase. So my hair won't be in my eyes, I put my hair in two little ponytails. I have a big bomber jacket that I wear with the *Christmas Spectacular* logo on it. Between my hair and my not wearing makeup, my mom is not pleased.

"Greta, I just don't get why you don't want to wear makeup. I mean, you're wearing your Rockette jacket and you're . . . you're just not put together."

"I don't want to wear makeup because it causes more acne!" I yell at her. The truth is, though, that she's right to a degree. I'm not put together. I'm a fucking mess. Maybe if I let her in on my secret that I'm contemplating suicide, instead of acting like my life is going so well during their visit, she would react differently.

All in all, we have a nice time. My family is impressed by the show. I know they are proud of me.

Not long after my mom's visit, my dad, my aunts, my uncles, and my cousins all come to see the show. My family loved the show and seemed proud of me. I feel excited and honored, but also embarrassed. I don't deserve the attention. *If only they knew what you do with food when they're not around!*

My dad is thrilled by the *Christmas Spectacular* show and how I'm able to perform all of the numbers. The little people especially intrigue him.

"They aren't midgets, they're little people," my dad corrects my cousin, after having been corrected by me.

I give my family a tour of the city and go to destination restaurants like Top of the Rock, John's Pizza, and we eat Italian food in Little Italy. I, of course, purge through all of my meals, but since it's second nature, it doesn't ruin my fun, it allows me to have fun.

By December, I start dreading going to work. I begin dreading everything. Depression consumes me. I dread going to my apartment because of the silent tension that exists in a home when one member—me—is consistently behind her locked bedroom door hunched over in her closet trying not to let the sound of puking in plastic bags or cups or whatever carry across the paper-thin walls into her roommates' bedroom. I haven't been to Michele's class nearly all season, which makes me dread going back because my consistent absence will leave me feeling out of the loop. *There's always someone in the sidelines waiting to replace you.*

I've had this feeling of dread before when I've worked in restaurants. It's hell to be a bulimic surrounded by trays of food. It's like a drug addict working in a restaurant where servers take mirrors piled with thick powdery lines of cocaine to table twelve and table forty-two, where patrons sit eagerly with their utensils—their razors, straws, and dollar bills—hungry to be high.

As a bulimic server, I'm not only irritated by the sensory stimuli,

I'm constantly reminded of the dearth of self. The craving to cork the bottomless pit of emptiness and the relentless psychic ache that gnaws at me, day after day, and never heals. It's a reminder of who I am: a food addict.

So, when I don't like my job at a restaurant, I simply stop going. My rationale for this is that when I don't want to go to work, I start craving to binge, which gives me the excuse not to go. I don't call in to say I'm sick or to give my two-week notice. I just don't go. One time, I walked out midshift, telling the restaurant manager that I'd started my period and had to run down the street to buy tampons. I never went back. My consequence for my behavior, besides the financial instability, is that I can never return as a patron to the restaurants I walk out of. I don't care. There are hundreds of restaurants in New York. Besides, I don't need to be eating out.

In the restaurant business, I've had probably fifty serving jobs over the years, and only a handful I've kept for more than three months. But with dance, I'd always shown up, despite any depressive or disordered state, as the embarrassment and consequences of pulling a no-show would be too great in the small circle of the dance business.

Toward the end of the season, on a frosty December morning, I wake up truly depressed and bloated from the previous night of bingeing and purging. Snow is falling outside my window. I don't want to go to work. I want to stay home in bed. I don't feel like putting on my full-length, wind-protected coat to travel in the snow from Astoria two stops on the subway into Manhattan. I don't want to feel uncomfortable in my tight costumes, or dance in the line with cliquey bitches who don't like me.

I weigh my options. I can't call in sick because I've already used up my sick days. Dancers don't just skip out on a gig like the Rockettes. I could be fired. On some level, I don't care. The worst part would be explaining my behavior to Sherry, my dance captain. I can't run away from the dance world like I do the restaurant world. There isn't another job down the street. Not to mention, I see these people in class.

I run my hand over my stomach to see just how fat I am. I'm so bloated. Thoughts of bacon, egg, cheese biscuits, and hash browns from McDonald's interrupt my inspection. There's a McDonald's one block away, on Thirtieth Avenue, the only food and shopping strip close to my Astoria abode.

Bingeing and purging won't alleviate my bloat immediately, but after one or two episodes of eating and emptying, enough time will pass that my stomach will feel flat again. *No, there's no way I can make it through the day at Radio City.* I know, by the way, just how irrational all of this is. But at this point, I've already done a grand jeté over the line, leaving behind my freedom to choose, and landing, toe-ball-heel, of course, onto the black-and-white concrete of rigidity. My only choice is to binge and purge.

With my decision made, I put on my coat, scarf, gloves, and boots, and head to McDonald's. I'll deal with my no-show, no-call later. Luckily, I deposited my weekly paycheck, so I have plenty of money. I earn more than $1,500 a week, but between my food expenses and bills, I'm practically broke by the time Friday hits. I can't get to McDonald's fast enough.

As a bulimic, there are days when I feel completely excited to binge, like a kid about to climb onto a ride at Disney World. Other days, I feel depressed, standing teary-eyed and confounded in the cookie aisle of the grocery store, wishing I could stop myself. Today, I feel a combination of excitement, fear, and guilt. I don't want to think about the aftermath. *What will I say to Sherry? What will she say to me? What will the other girls think?* It's all pretty embarrassing. I'll deal with it later. For now, all I have to think about is which and how many extra-value breakfast meals I want to buy.

After I get my large bag of breakfast food, I stop into the Italian market for some fresh mozzarella. I've never been inside before, but the huge balls of creamy white mozzarella always catch my eye as I pass by the window storefront; today seems as good a time as any to have one. Immediately after exiting the shop, I dig my house key into the durable protective plastic around the mozzarella ball to free the cheese. The denseness of it looks delicious. With my bag in one hand and my ball in the other, I'm starting to forget about what I've done. I begin to enjoy my morning. As I walk, I pull long strips of mozzarella and pop them into my mouth, as if I'm eating Laffy Taffy. People stare at me as I pass by them eating the softball of cheese. I imagine pitching the ball of cheese in between their judgmental pair of eyes, but decide it's too good to waste on an asshole. As if it's not normal to be eating mozzarella on a snowy public sidewalk. I consume half of the two-pound ball before arriving home.

I walk up the stairwell to my second floor apartment and go directly to my room. My roommates will most likely be sleeping all day, since they decided to roll on Ecstasy last night, a plus for me. I peel off my gloves, unravel the scarf hugging my neck, throw my coat on the bed, and kick off my snowy boots. I've had enough mozzarella for the time being, so I set it on my nightstand and dig into the fast-food bag. I eat a breakfast burrito, three hash browns, one cinnamon roll, two strips of bacon, an egg and cheese biscuit, and one large Diet Coke, light ice. I have more food in my bag, but my stomach can't hold any more for now. Once I hit around the 1,500-calorie mark, I have to throw up.

I grab a hair tie, put my hair up in a ponytail, and grab a plastic bag. I go into my closet, holding the bag with one hand, lean over and put my free hand under my stomach. I don't stick my finger down my throat. I haven't done that in years. I have a technique where I push on my stomach in a certain way just below my belly button, and I flex my abs, a one-two motion that thrusts any food I have eaten up and out of my body.

Knowing that purging McDonald's biscuits and cinnamon rolls is about as easy as running uphill in a knee-high pool of mud, I drink extra soda to ease the possible stress on my esophagus. *Because I care so much about myself.* I lean over to do my one-two, heave-ho, as I do every day. The first couple of thrusts go fine, relieved that my breakfast is in the plastic bag instead of digesting in my stomach. I lean over once more. As I flex my abs, triggering the food to come up, something doesn't feel right on my insides. I feel like something is stuck inside of my esophagus.

Beginning to panic, I thrust my stomach harder. Oh . . . my . . . God! The rush of anxiety flushes my face. I'm . . . I'm . . . I'm choking. I'm choking! Fucking hell, I'm choking on the strings of the mozzarella cheese! I can feel them stuck in my throat. Envisioning the organ or rib it must be coiled around. I thrust my stomach again, until I can feel the long snake of a piece slither up, peering out of the back of my throat. I drop the plastic bag full of puke, shove my hand down my throat, and start pulling the stuck piece out of my body. It's not working! *Why, why, why did you have to get the God damn mozzarella! If you had just gone to work! You stupid idiot. Why do you keep doing this to yourself? What's wrong with you?* With both hands now, I'm pulling on the mozzarella, playing tug-a-rope with my innards. Finally, it comes out.

Jeez-us! That was a close call. My insides, my outsides, I'm a bundle of nerves. I easily could've choked to death. I can see the headlines now, "Death by Mozzarella Ball: A Bulimic's Worst Nightmare." A headline possibly dazzling enough to make *The New York Times.* I peek into my McDonald's bag to see the remaining food. Agh, I don't want anymore. I'm finished for today, having scared myself silly.

I clean up my mess and take my bags outside to the trash can. On my way back inside, I hear my phone ringing. I cringe knowing who it's going to be.

"Beeeeeep! You have one message," the answering machine blares. "Hi, Greta, it's Sherry. We are all extremely worried about you. I'm wondering where you are and if you're coming today. I just want to know that you're okay. Please call me as soon as you receive this message."

I have dreaded this inevitable phone call all morning. There's no more getting lost in my fast-food frenzy or distracting myself with that sinister and sneaky mozzarella. Over the next hour, Sherry calls me three more times. Reality begins to set. She's expecting me to call her back. Although I don't feel ready to, I know, soon enough, I'll have to face the music.

I know by my apathy and choice to binge instead of go to work as a Rockette, I am in the midst of my own great wooden soldier fall. The momentum is picking up, my behavior pushing the limits and speeding up the consequences. Will anyone catch me? Will this soldier be able to pop back up and smile at the audience after surviving?

It's too early to tell.

You Have Only Two Options

O nce out of mozzarella hell, I again listen to the message Sherry left me. No, there is no way I can call her. What am I going to tell her? *Hi, Sherry. Sorry I couldn't make it today. I was too busy shoving extra value meals down my throat and choking on mozzarella to call you.* I'm totally fucked. Getting fired would be the best outcome as I see it, because the thought of facing everyone, the thought of walking into that dressing room to see the dancers' critical glances—and know they are whispering about me behind the costume racks—feels intolerable.

Not showing up today was one of my biggest blunders yet. Sure, I had quit at least thirty jobs in the past because I chose to act out my eating disorder instead of fulfill my responsibilities. But those were restaurant jobs. Jobs I cared nothing about. Not showing up to Radio City is another story. As I replay the last few hours and the decision to risk a job I've dreamed of having, I know that this is the progression I hear so much about in the rooms of Overeaters Anonymous.

I pick up the phone, my index finger hoping to push the numbers in just the right way to reach Sherry's voicemail.

"Hello, this is Sherry."

"It's . . . it's Greta. I'm, I'm so sorry that I didn't show up today."

"I was so worried. Where were you? What happened?" Sherry asked.

"Well . . . you see . . . it's just that . . . I, I have this problem." That's a good start.

"What type of problem, Greta?" Sherry asked.

"I have an eating disorder. I'm bulimic." There. I said it.

"Oh my God, Greta," Sherry said. "I had no idea. How long has this been going on?"

"Well, it's really been bad lately. I've had it since I was sixteen. It started kind of like a diet, and then just got really out of control."

"I'm so sorry, Greta. I wish you would've called me and told me what was going on."

"I was embarrassed. It's not really the type of thing you want your dance captain to know about. I didn't want any of the dancers to know. Well, except Heather—she knows. She's tried to help me through the season, but I've just been so depressed that it's gotten worse." I feel like ten pounds have been lifted off of my chest. *Too bad it's not your ass.*

Unexpectedly, Sherry opens up. "A few years ago, my husband and I were having a lot of problems and I thought we were going to get divorced. We ended up going to therapy and spiritual counseling. We're really into our church. It helped us a lot. It was a really difficult time for me. I was really depressed."

"Thanks for sharing that with me, Sherry. That must've been really hard. How did you get through it?" I couldn't believe what I was hearing. Not only was Sherry identifying with me, but she understood me, at least to some degree. This isn't the outcome I expected.

"It was our pastor that helped the most. And we went to counseling for quite a while." The word pastor has always flipped my stomach. I hope Sherry doesn't tell me to go to church and pray about it.

"So, what will happen to me for not showing up?" Here it is. Doomsday.

"Well, Greta. I've actually not had this issue come up before. It's the end of the season. Do you think you will be able to return for the last week of shows?"

"Yes, for sure I will be there." I didn't want to go back. Even though Sherry is being supportive, I'm not so sure I can trust her. I want to, but dancers can be so two-faced.

"Well, then I'll just see you back next week." Sherry said.

Streams of salt pour down my cheeks the second I hang up the phone. I'm pathetic. I stand up from the couch, tighten my fist, and punch myself as hard as I can in the stomach. I deserve it. I keep punching myself until my stomach can't take another blow. Couldn't I have just waited one more week for the season to end?

The following week, I stand at the Stage Door entrance of the Music Hall—the place I was sure would be the beginning of a better, bulimia-free life. I can't believe it is the last week of the season. I had so many aspirations: I was going to save money, treat myself and my body well, not let my insecurities set me apart from the other cast members. I was going to experience New York and, for once, not let my eating disorder ruin every experience. None of my goals have been met. I didn't change my life. The only change is that my behavior has gotten worse, I've gained weight, I'm more depressed, and I have attained new levels of self-hatred.

It's so confusing. Even with this job, I can't see my worth. Intellectually, I know that to become a Rockette in New York is ridiculously competitive. I should be thrilled just to have the chance, which I am. But when am I going to get it? When will I finally feel that I am worth enough? When will I stop trying to kill myself through this slow torture?

I exit the elevator and walk into the dressing room. Dancers' eyes shift in my direction, their lips turning upward to say hello to me before focusing back on themselves in the mirror or on the costume racks. So far, no one has tried to humiliate me with shouts of *psycho* or *bulimic freak* or *no-talented-fat-fuck* character assaults that I've imagined. It is business as usual up here on the fifth floor. Maybe Sherry didn't tell anyone anything.

"Are you okay?" Heather asks. "I was really worried about you when you didn't show up." Heather is the only dancer in the cast that knows the depth of my struggle.

"Yeah, I'm alright. The eating disorder is out of control."

Heather and I became friends instantly because we were assigned to sit next to each other in the dressing room. On the first day of rehearsal when we all ran to see our dressing-table assignments, I realized as fast as a thirty-second quick change that my dressing area signified my low-level status in the New York production. Heather and I were next to the dressing room door and isolated from the rest of the cast. It's like being seated at a table next to the busy kitchen at Il Mulino restaurant, nowhere near the chef.

"How was last week?" I ask, moving on from my drama. Heather takes my lead and starts talking about Sherry's notes from the last show.

I sit down at my dressing table. I'm feeling less nervous since no one brought up my unacceptable behavior. I look at myself in the mirror. *Don't berate yourself today. For once, try to be good to yourself.* Out of the corner of my eye, I see them hanging on the costume rack. I despise them. The sparkle tights and green velvet costume has become my nemesis. Every time I put on this ensemble, I feel like I'm in an episode of *Montel Williams* where a skinny teenager who previously made fun of fat people has volunteered to put on a fat suit, to see how it physically and emotionally feels to be heavy and ostracized by society. Later she recounts on national television how horrible it felt and how she will never make fun of fat people again. *Until next week when the cameras aren't rolling.* The difference between me and the girl posing as a fat person is that the only person making fun of me is me.

I roll my two pairs of tights on and step into the dreaded green blob of a costume.

"Heather," I say, "Can you zip me up, please?" The higher the zipper crawls up my spine, the tighter the costume gets and the more constriction I feel. I can barely stand to have underwear touch my skin when I feel fat. Putting this green velvet fat suit on top of the ten pounds I've gained is almost unbearable. My fat needs to breathe! *I can't stand this. I will not be able to get through this. Leave now. Just leave. No, you can't leave. Just get through today. You can binge and purge when you get home.* Food is my only salvation.

FOLLOWING MY NEAR-DEATH experience with a cheese ball, I decide to be serious. The season at Radio City is over, which allows me more time to attend meetings. I acquire a food sponsor, which means that I call in my food to a person every morning so that I'm accountable. Something has to change.

I make connections with people at the meetings. Soon, I have forty-five days of abstinence put together. I'm lying to myself. I did what I call a quick-purge on day twenty-nine, but I'm not going to count it. I can't go back to day one again. So, I don't.

My friend Scarlett also attends Overeaters Anonymous meetings. We met a couple of years ago when I was in a period of abstinent eating and I agreed to be her food sponsor. Now though, Scarlett and I are in the same boat. We dip our feet into the waters of recovery for a minute or two, collecting eighteen days of abstinent time here, forty-two days there, but then decide the tide is too rough to swim in and retreat to our sugary shore of safety and security.

Scarlett is the type of Upper East Side mother I idolize. She's 5'10" with shimmering green eyes. She likes to remind me, "Everyone always says I have hair and eyebrows like Brooke Shields." She can't weigh more than 110 pounds. Her husband, Sean, is a corporate bigwig at Armani, which means that Scarlett can stay home with her son, Carson, who watches *Thomas the Train* DVDs for hours or has play dates with the neighbors' children, while she obsesses over when she can next eat her fat-free turkey and mustard sandwich half.

At the end of the meeting one Wednesday evening, a girl named Vivian announces she needs a roommate. Vivian has five years of sobriety and over one year of no bingeing and purging. Something that is hard for me to imagine ever having.

The thought of living in the city is amazing. No more lonely Astoria nights bingeing on pancakes at the Star Greek diner. Meetings and my dance classes would be at my fingertips. There'd be no excuse to relapse. I've seen Vivian at these meetings for several months now. We say hello and smile, but nothing more. After the meeting, I walk over to her.

"Vivian, right?" I said.

"Yes. You're Greta?" It's like the first day of school. I'm hoping she won't judge me on my short period of abstinence.

"I'm really interested in moving to the city. How much is the rent?" I ask.

"Oh, great. I really need someone. The rent is $800." Whoa, that's pretty steep for me. Right now, I pay $600, and I can barely afford that with all of the money I spend on food. But I reason (lie to myself) that if I'm in the city, then I'll be happier and less prone to bingeing. I may even be able to save money. Yes, this will be a great move.

"When do you need someone by?" I ask.

"Two weeks." Oh, boy. That will be tough.

"Oh, okay. I think I can do that." I have no idea how I will be able to pull this together in two weeks. I don't have a lot of money because I just started a new serving job, but I can get the security deposit back from my roommate and try to earn the rest of the money by working extra shifts at the restaurant. I have to make this work. It is my only way to food freedom. This is how I make all financial decisions. Rationalization and denial—two defenses I have mastered.

"And how much time do you have?" Vivian asks, referring to my abstinence.

"Forty-five days . . . but, it was just a slip. I've had much longer periods of abstinence in the past." Lying was the only chance I had of securing a room in Manhattan.

"Well, as long as you're going to meetings," she says. Her eyes say she's not too sure about me, but she ignores her intuition.

"Oh, yes, I go all the time." I go all of the time and still relapse is what I should've said.

Taking the train back to Astoria, I think about how I will break the news to Marcy. More importantly, I have to think of how I will get my half of the security deposit back.

The next morning, I wake up, dreading the conversation I know I have to have. I walk into the kitchen. Marcy is making coffee.

"How was your night?" I ask.

"Fine. Bobby and I just went to a club." They were always going to clubs. Drinking, rolling, smoking. I've always been uncomfortable around Bobby. Maybe it's because I know Marcy's parents don't like Bobby. They are worried about her eating disorder and her relationship. Yes, Marcy has an eating disorder, but not one as serious as mine. Hers is more like an adolescent phase. The type that my parents had hoped I had.

Marcy and Bobby and I have an unspoken rule about my eating disorder: No one is allowed to discuss it. I binge and purge in the privacy of my room and they say nothing. But, like all of the other roommates, our denial creates uneasiness.

"I wanted to let you know that I am moving out. I have a chance to live in the city. And I think I need to so that I can be close to my Overeaters Anonymous meetings." I can always use the eating disorder as a crutch.

"Well, how am I going to pay for this apartment?"

"You have a good serving job. And Bobby works. You will be able to handle it fine, I'm sure." Marcy is working at an Asian restaurant in Times Square. I told her about the job because I worked for their Uptown location. She makes great money.

She's pissed. I thought she'd be happy.

Ten days later with all of my belongings in cardboard boxes I see the money sitting on the kitchen counter. Thank God. I grab my backpack and a couple of boxes, heading toward the subway. It takes me multiple trips, but I don't care. I'm just glad to have a Manhattan zip code. Vivian buzzes me up to my new apartment. I hike up the five flights. *Hey, maybe this will help me lose weight.*

"Knock, knock, knock," I say.

"Hi! Come in, come in." Vivian is excited to see me. Vivian's place is typical of a New York City apartment. Exposed brick walls, books and knick-knacks cluttered in crevices, a window unit air conditioner, and an ancient kitchen. A large antique rug covered with cat hair is center on the living room floor. I grew up with large dogs. I hate cats.

"Thanks!" I say. "So, my bed, dresser, television, and chair will arrive tomorrow."

"Great. I thought we could put your chair next to mine, right here," Vivian says, motioning toward the identical Papasan chair we both have from Pier 1 Imports.

"Sounds great. Thanks again for letting me move in. Oh, and, here's the deposit money."

Marcy left me only half of the security, so I have to pull the rest from my bank account. Now I am left with practically nothing. Even though I have been abstinent for the greater part of six weeks, I'm behind from the financial damage of earlier bingeing episodes. I'm in constant financial hardship, regularly having to explain to my mother why my phone is turned off. And now, I've decided to move into an apartment where I pay $200 more a month. *Brilliant idea.*

"Oh, thanks," she says, as I hand her every cent to my name. "You can have the bedroom. I always fall asleep watching television on the futon in the living room."

Wow, I can't believe I am here. I have wanted to be back in the city forever! I race to the window in my new room. Nice view. I love the grit and grime of First Avenue. Something about the smell of the city makes me feel more alive.

"Well, I'm about to go to the lunch-time meeting at Ramaz, so I'm going to head out," Vivian says.

I should probably be going to the meeting, too, but I'll make another meeting. If not today, then tomorrow. I have no desire to binge and purge.

I'M NOT MAKING enough money at my current restaurant, so I quit and start working at a popular pizzeria on the Upper East Side. My friend Jonathon is the manager. I know him from my Tremaine dancing days in Hollywood. He also takes classes from my teacher Michele. Within a week of working, I have a love interest. Her name is Erica, a short black-haired Jewish girl who's planning to backpack through Europe in a couple of months. Erica and I flirt back and forth. We drink rum and cokes (diet for me, of course), get drunk, make out on the soot-filled rooftop of her sixth-floor walkup, and fall asleep together.

Every time, I sneak out before seven in the morning.

"You're making me feel cheap," she says one morning.

"Sorry, it's not you. I just am an early-morning person. I like to get up and get out of the house." The truth is that I feel too ashamed about and uncomfortable being with a woman. I keep telling myself that I don't really like it; it's just because I am drunk.

Every time there is a pizza mistake in the kitchen, the employees can eat it. At least once per shift, I stand with Pablo, the dishwasher, shoving thin slices of pepperoni or sausage pizza into my mouth. After which, I drink several mouthfuls of Diet Coke, and then go straight to the bathroom. It isn't long before my friend and manager Jonathon notices my behavior.

"Greta, can you come in the office?" Jonathon asks, at the end of my shift one evening.

"Is everything okay," I say. Embarrassment is already flooding my face. I know exactly what is coming.

"Greta, it's your eating. You spend most of your time eating the pizza mistakes in the kitchen."

"I know, but we're allowed to do that. I always do my job well."

"Greta, let's be honest. I know you are eating and throwing up."

"Well, that might be true, but I'm still doing an adequate job." I'm totally pissed. He is completely using our past dealings against me. When Jonathon and I were both on scholarship at Tremaine Dance Center in Los Angeles, I made some snide and immature remarks about him. I didn't even mean them. I was just trying to impress Natasha, the first girl I ever had a crush on. Clearly, he hasn't let it go and is using it and my personal weakness against me. *Queenie Bitch.*

"Greta, you simply aren't focused. I know we've been friends, but I'm your manager. You need to get it together, or you can't work here." *Pompous prick.*

"Okay, I got it. Can I go now?" I fight back tears. I was shocked, but it wasn't the first time I've been reprimanded by restaurant management for eating. When I worked at a Mexican restaurant in Greenwich Village, the manager would threaten my job every time he saw me eating tortilla chips. In Los Angeles, I worked at an ice cream shop and would get in trouble for eating too many samples in between customers. In Kansas, I ate and purged my way through all of my shifts at a diner. I mean, really, what's a bulimic server supposed to do when there are pancakes, macaroni and cheese, and chili fries on the menu?

I'm also relapsing at home, something I told Vivian I'd never do. More than just relapsing, I'm using (stealing) my mom's, dad's, and Kent's credit card numbers to order food deliveries—something I haven't done since I lived in Los Angeles. At one time or another, they have each trusted me with their credit card numbers to purchase airline tickets. I saved them for future use.

Since I spend all of my money on food and quit my jobs regularly, the credit card numbers are my only saving grace. When my parents check their credit card bills and freak out over the charges for thousands of dollars of New York City food deliveries, my only other option is to pawn my (or anyone else's) CDs at a thrift store or to pawn my jewelry in the Diamond District.

I walk into the lobby of an Upper East Side prewar apartment building and buzz 1-C, the new office of my therapist Heather. My hand pulls open the door when I feel the doorknob vibrate, signaling that I'm sane enough to enter. Recounting my behaviors over the last couple of weeks and months, hell, years, I'm not so sure I'm sane at all. The doorman is not at his post this morning. Usually, we exchange our weekly smiles as I make a beeline for Heather's office. I try not to look like a patient. *Don't worry, Mister, I have it all together.*

I walk through the door, trying to avoid the floor-to-ceiling mirror, but am not strong enough to turn away. My life stops. The mirror has taken me hostage. Self-torture fills me as I take my usual inventory—waist, butt, thighs, arms. *Love handles, big ass, wide legs, thick arms.* I try to stop myself from scolding other body parts, but my eyes are forced to look at my face. *Disgusting. Big nose, pitted cheeks. The only thing you have going for you are your blue eyes. If they were brown, it's possible you would be one of the ugliest people on the planet.*

The waiting room of Heather's office is typical. Two chairs, tranquil pictures hanging on the wall, and a small rectangular table with a radio sitting on the bottom shelf playing classical music. In front of Heather's office door is a sound machine that blocks out any patient rants or sobs that Bach and Chopin cannot. Waiting, I gaze anxiously outside at nearby dreary brown brick apartment buildings.

Heather opens the door.

"Hi, Greta. I'll be right with you," she says, almost in a whisper. "I'm just going to use the washroom." I don't know much about Heather's upbringing, but the fact that she says washroom and not bathroom, or "rezource" instead of resource, makes me think she's of a different class than I am.

I look up from the book I'm reading to make her think that I'm not waiting for her, to make her think that my life really does not revolve around the fifty-five minutes I feel safe in her office.

"You can come in, Greta," Heather says, as she exits the washroom. I stand up from my chair in a purposeful way, suck in my stomach, and stand at a diagonal angle, trying to appear skinnier than the fat bitch in the lobby mirror minutes earlier. I know it's no use, not today.

Heather's office is a big box. The scent of Joe Malone's Lime Basil perfume floats around the room. Her black leather chair sits diagonally across from my seat, the patient couch that hugs my back as I sink into it. We both sit in our assigned spots. Her office has become my sanctuary, the only place I feel safe from myself and the world. Once seated, I cross my legs the way I was taught to do in Rockettes, not allowing the top leg to put the full weight of itself on the bottom leg, which results in a thinner line. I angle my knees so that they are perfectly opposite of Heather. I don't want her to see the full fatty width of the thigh that's being smashed by my other leg.

Heather's walls are dressed with diplomas from Columbia University, New York University, and The New School—all schools I dream to go to when I eventually return to school. I never noticed them in her other office. *Wow. I could never be accepted into those schools.* Behind Heather's chair stands a bookshelf filled with books on therapy and self-help. I scan the titles, *The Dance of Anger, Object Relations,* and *Codependent No More,* making mental notes of books I may need for my clinical library collection in the future.

I've known since the age of sixteen that I will be a therapist when I stop dancing, if my eating disorder doesn't kill me first. Besides dancing, eating disorders and addiction are the only things I'm well versed in. I don't know yet that ten years later I will be sitting in Heather's office telling her of my acceptances into all of the schools she has diplomas from, or that I will have a collection of professional therapy books at home on my bookshelf.

I've been seeing Heather for many months now. Heather is almost eleven years older than me, although if she wore her hair in a ponytail I bet she would still be carded for alcohol. Sometimes she wears glasses, but today she doesn't. She's in her athletic pants and T-shirt, which tells me she will be going or already has gone to Equinox Fitness.

I try to squeeze as much personal information out of Heather as possible. Before she will give me anything, we always have to have a therapeutic dialogue about it.

Heather is the current person I have picked to be the savior of my life. Given my fragile emotional state, she recently gave me her cell phone and her home phone number to use if I'm in a desperate situation. Not only does this allowance give me a feeling that I am more significant in her life than her other patients, but it gives me a feeling that I'm significant as a human being. I'm sure she doesn't really want me to use them, so I feel badly every time I dial her number. *Needy bitch.*

Heather sits down and looks at me. Her smile is full of warmth and empathy as she scans my face, looking deep into my eyes with intent.

"How are you, Greta?" She doesn't miss a beat. She can already tell that I'm in a bad space. I'm already thinking that in fifty-four minutes I'll be thrown out of her office, just one in a caseload of patients she has.

"I'm okay, I guess."

"You don't look okay. You look depressed. What's going on?"

"Well, my manager at the pizzeria called me into his office and confronted me about my eating disorder." I can't make eye contact with Heather.

"What? What did he say?" I tell her the whole story, streaming tears of embarrassment down my cheeks.

"That is totally inappropriate that he did that, Greta. That's fucked up." For a second, I want to smile hearing Heather curse at Jonathon, but then I segue into eating disorder dialogue.

"And I'm gaining weight. I'm trying to eat on a food plan, but then I also binge and purge. And sometimes I'm so depressed that I don't purge. I just punish myself by keeping the food in my stomach. I'm not going to dance classes because I'm so fat and too embarrassed. I . . . I just hate myself. Sometimes I just want to die."

Heather explores my statement about wanting to die by doing a quick suicide risk assessment before allowing me to continue.

"No, I don't have any plans to hurt myself. You don't have to call the police." *Although, maybe you will need to in the future.* "I just can't get out of it. I went to the grocery store, stood in the cereal aisle, and started crying. I didn't want to binge, but I had to. It just isn't getting any better."

"You're having a hard time making eye contact with me today, Greta," Heather says.

"I know," I say, my eyes finding the courage to look at her before looking down again. "I just feel ashamed."

"Uh huh. You poor lamb." I sit and cry with Heather for a few moments, before pushing the uncomfortable emotions back down.

"One good thing is that I got a job at the Lenox Room as a cocktail server," I say.

I look down at my cell phone. Ten minutes left. Anxiety starts to build.

"What's going on with you right now, Greta?" Heather's so perceptive.

"It's almost time to go." Fear is pushing tears to the surface. "I don't want to go out there," I say, motioning to the door. "I don't want to go out into the world. This is the only place I feel safe." Now the water works are on full blast. As if I'm back in first grade being dropped off at my new school for the first time.

Heather looks at me lovingly. My heart is aching. I don't want to face the world. How will I survive until I see Heather next week? How will I feel nurtured?

"Greta, it is scary to go out in the world sometimes."

"This hour is the only time I feel like I get my emotional needs met. I almost don't even want it, because it hurts. It physically hurts. Knowing the feeling and then having to let go of it gives me this gnawing."

"Uh-huh. You know, Greta, you don't have to leave our relationship here. You can carry it with you wherever you go. It's like putting me in your pocket. When you feel unsafe, you can think of our work. You can know that I'm here for you. You can always call me if you need to."

"Okay."

"Well, Greta. Our time is up, I'm afraid." Heather and I stand up, do our end-of-the-session hug. "You are going to be just fine, Greta. I know you can do it." I nod yes. Maybe I can.

The following day, I start my new job. I work one shift at the Lenox room and decide it's not for me. The truth is that I'm left-handed, and whenever I'm asked to open a wine bottle, I flashback to a terrible experience opening a wine bottle when I was sixteen years old, and I've avoided it ever since. So I quit. I'm not worried. There is no shortage of restaurant jobs in NYC.

A week later, I start training for a new job at the Greenwich Café. Within minutes of scanning over the menu and watching the way the manager rants, I know this job's not for me. I have to get out somehow. As soon as the manager says I have to work five training shifts without pay, I start devising an exit plan. Rather than say it's not a good fit, I make up something.

"Uh, Miranda," I say to my trainer. "I . . . this is so embarrassing, but I just started my period. I have to go to Duane Reade or CVS and buy some tampons."

"Oh, I have one you can have."

"Uh, I better buy some. I'm really heavy my first day. I'll be right back." And with that, I was off. I passed Greenwich Avenue and headed toward the Donut Pub for a fresh baker's dozen.

Now I have no job and I spend at least $50 a day on binge food. My money is quickly disappearing. I don't want to, but I have to make a phone call to my mother to ask her for money. I'm dreading the call. I hate doing this. I have to ask frequently because it's impossible to keep up with my bingeing and purging.

"Hi, Mommy. How are you?" I'm trying to mask the familiar tone of my voice that precludes begging my mom for money.

"Hi, Greta." I can tell from her tone of voice that she is irritated.

"Greta, you used Kent's credit card again! I told you not to use it!!" I knew that was coming. I don't want to use his card numbers, but when I'm desperate, I'm desperate.

"I know, I'm sorry." There's nothing I can really say.

"God, how much are you eating, Greta? I thought your eating was getting better."

"I don't know . . . it's not getting better."

"Are you even dancing anymore?"

"Yes, I still take Michele's class." I lied. I hadn't been to Michele's class in over a month. I had gained ten pounds and was too embarrassed and depressed to return.

"Hmm. Well, you've got to figure out how to get yourself together, Greta. You need to discipline yourself."

"I know."

"So how's work? You're still at the Lenox Room?"

"Uh, no. I didn't like it."

"So, how are you going to pay your bills?"

"Well, I have another job. A café in the Village. But I'm still in training."

"Uh-huh." My mother is not interested at this point in hearing about my financial woes.

"Mommy, do you think you can send me some money?" I got it out.

"God damn it, Greta. You have got to get a handle on your finances!"

"I know!"

"Yeah, I'll Western Union it. How much do you need?" I hate this question. As much as possible would be accurate.

"I guess $500," I say, lowering my voice.

"Fine. But Greta, you have to figure this out."

"I know. Thanks, Mommy." *I'm such an asshole.* If parenting skills were based on monetary donations, both my mom and dad would win Parent of the Year awards.

The following day, I pick up my money, vowing to myself that I will not use it to binge. Of course, within hours I am at the grocery store.

Later that day, I'm hired for a job at the Mustang Grill, a Mexican restaurant on the Upper East Side. I start eating and purging my way through the shifts. Scarlett and I hang out there after work, but I quit the job one month later because I can't stop bingeing and purging.

I binge my way through the hundreds of dollars my mom and dad have each sent me, until I'm once again out of money. As a last resort, I call Grandma Patty. I know she is on a fixed income, but I'm desperate. She sends me $400 and tells me she's happy to help. Wracked with guilt, I use the only resource I have, but am not allowed to use—my parents' credit cards—to eat away my shameful feelings.

I continue to go to therapy, even though I have no money. Heather has been nice enough to let me see her without paying her. "I know you will give me the money when you have it." I knew that I would, too.

Vivian just kicked me out of her apartment. She just confronted me, telling me that she knows I have not been abstinent while living with her. Not knowing what else to do with myself, I walk to Janus on Seventy-Fourth Street, the church that holds my favorite Overeaters Anonymous meeting. On the way to the meeting, I fail to notice the beautifully tree-lined streets or to admire the townhouses that I envision myself living in as I do every other time I walk to Janus. An apathetic taupe tarnishes my world. My bemusement for why and how my behavior landed me an eviction notice blinds any existing beauty.

I just don't get how I ended up here. Every single day, I plan exactly what I'm going to eat, I go to meetings, and I have fellowship with friends from the program. Yet on most days by midmorning, I'm already hugging the toilet. I keep thinking that one day I'll just get sick of eating. I fantasize about the final binge and purge that will push me over the edge into healthful eating. In between my jarfuls of peanut butter and jelly, I keep waiting to be struck abstinent, but that day never comes.

You people have it easy, I think to myself, looking into the eyes of the seemingly clear-minded people who pass me on the sidewalk. I reach into my purse, take a Camel Special Lights cigarette out, and light up. I take a long inhale, hearing the crackle as the carcinogenic filter burns. "Life sucks and then you die," I mumble to myself, letting out a smoky exhale. Such an appropriate phrase for my mood. I should probably start picking out my burial plot and headstone. *Poor me. Poor little ole me.*

I schlep my electrolyte-imbalanced body up the rickety flight of stairs and open the door to the meeting. The emaciated anorexics, the chipmunk-cheeked bulimics, and the lumpy, codependent-shuffling compulsive overeaters are all present. The familiar mixtures of insecure and blissful faces circle the room atop bodies crammed next to one another on folding chairs, donated spongy couches, and the piano bench. Some bony butts are even sitting on the floor.

I can always tell who's having bad body image by the way they sit—legs crossed tightly like a Twizzler candy, arms folded, forty-year-olds with wrinkled foreheads and angry eyebrows—all looking as though they're still suffering from teenage angst.

The Wednesday night meeting always packs in a full house because of its anorexic-bulimic focus, which allows all of us who are anorexic and bulimic—the much-preferred disorders to have over the gluttonous compulsive overeater disorder—to have both the visual and cognitive acuity that we aren't as freakish as we feel. I tiptoe daintily across the floor trying hard not to step on any overfed fingers or withered limbs as I make my way to Scarlett, who gives me the hand signal to sit next to her.

Almost daily, Scarlett and I hang out at her brownstone. We stand in her French Provencal kitchen savoring our 160-calorie pints of the controversial Tasti D-Lite frozen dessert, while incessantly talking about how our lives will be so much better when we can stop throwing up. We sit politely in the bars of swank Upper East Side restaurants, sipping our glasses of pinot noir, while we make grandiose plans to open a children's hair salon "when we're well," because you know, these days, you can charge $25 for a kid's haircut. Neither of us has a degree in cosmetology, nor plans to pursue one.

I squeeze myself in between Scarlett and a newcomer.

"Are you okay?" Scarlett whispers. "You look like you've been crying."

"It's a long story," I say. "I'll tell you after the meeting." She smiles at me sincerely and gives my arm a set of comforting pity pats. *Yes, isn't it awful? You haven't even heard my story and you know how tragic it must be. Poor me.*

Tracy, the leader of the meeting, spouts with her gratitude-filled smile, "Would anyone like to share their day counts?"

Since I've come into the Overeaters Anonymous rooms in the city, I've been obsessed with counting my days of abstinence. After every relapse, and there are too many to count, I test myself to see how long I will go until the next dreaded binge and purge episode. People begin to raise their hands.

"Hi, my name is Lacey and I'm an anorexic bulimic. I have forty-seven days of abstinence." Everyone claps.

"Dennis is next," Tracy calls out, "followed by Julie and then Michael."

"Hi, my name is Dennis, I'm a food addict, and I have 106 days off of sugar." More clapping. "I can't even believe it has been almost four months since my last binge. As most of you know, I used to eat dozens of those darn Krispy Kremes, cardboard box and all."

Dennis is a sixty-something food addict who, at almost every meeting, uses his obsession with the sinfully sweet glazed donuts as a point of reference to remember where he came from. The room reacts with a cool ha, ha, ha under our breaths every time he says this. No one is ever quite sure if he's kidding about eating the cardboard box. Never put it past a food addict.

I feel like waving my arms around in the air and shouting out to the room, "Hey, everybody, I'm at day zero, anyone want to clap for me?"

After everyone who wants to volunteer shares their day counts, Tracy speaks up. "Does anyone have one year or multiples thereof?"

A bright-eyed blond shoots her hand upward. "Hi, my name is Julie, I'm an anorexic, and I had five years on Saturday!"

Enthusiastic echoes of "All right!" and "You go, girl!" flutter around the room.

"Tell us, Julie, how'd you do it?"

Silence greets the room. The only audible movement comes from the crying ambulances outside heading to Gracie Square Hospital around the corner. All eyes are fixated on Julie, each eager to hear her response.

"It took me twelve years in this program to get *one* year of abstinence. And now I can't believe that I have five!" *Twelve years. Is she serious? How could it take her that long? That certainly won't be me.* "I also have to thank my sponsor because she was gracious enough to listen to my insanity, day after day. But the real person who saved me was my HP—my Higher Power. Without him, I could never have made it through, one day at a time."

Higher Power schmower. Whenever people talk about their HP as if *he's* their best friend or some other tangible being, I cringe. Higher Power—the omniscient being that grabbed the starring role in the *Big Book* of Alcoholics Anonymous—is usually attached to phrases like, "We have a spiritual problem," of which, our "only option" is to seek a "spiritual solution." *Sure. Right.*

Even as my cynical ears try to negate the pronouncements made by these proud, former pie-eating-pie-denying-pie-puking souls about how the program works—while I sit back and try to ignore the fact that I've just been kicked out of my apartment because of the excellent job I'm doing in handling recovery my own way—I know that they are right. I, too, have expressed the same praises of the program, becoming the Overeaters Anonymous cheerleader in my own abstinent glimpses.

"Okay. Would anyone like to bring up a topic for discussion?" I consider bringing up the topic of relapse, self-will, or hopelessness—all topics I am experiencing in this very moment—but instead clam up.

I'm too pissed at myself, and the world, to speak today.

I CALL HEATHER to come in for an emergency session.

"Vivian kicked me out. My eating sucks, I can't stop puking, I hate myself."

"Oh, no, Greta. I'm sorry to hear you're in such a bad spot."

I owe Heather money at this point because I binge and purge all the time.

"What is that on your arm?"

"A cut." I had worn my sleeves up on purpose that day, knowing what an observant person she is. I wanted her to see it. I hate myself for wanting her to see it.

"Greta, how did you cut yourself?"

"With a knife." After telling Heather more about cutting, my constant bingeing and purging, my feelings of self-loathing, and wanting to die, she says something that terrifies me.

"I feel powerless," Heather says. Shit. My savior is powerless. Now what the hell am I going to do? I knew, though, that she was powerless. When the eating disorder has progressed to this level, going to therapy once or twice a week will not alleviate the symptoms, no matter how brilliant the clinician.

"Greta, we need to figure out a plan. You are going to die if you don't go into treatment," Heather says.

"I know," I said. "I want to die."

After doing another quick suicidal risk assessment to be sure I'm not going to actually kill myself, Heather poses the question that I knew was coming.

"Do you want me to call your mom and Kent?" I don't want her to, but I need her to.

A couple of days later, I see my mom's phone number on my caller ID. It isn't Sunday, our assigned day to talk, so I'm guessing Heather called them. Even though I know we will soon have to discuss what I am going to do about my eating, I dread any conversation about it. I decide to let the voicemail answer so I can gauge her mood. My heart races as I press play on my phone.

"Oh, hi, Greta. We got a call from Heather. So . . . call me when you can." Her tone was warm. Much different from the annoyed tone she has had over the last several months when I'm begging her for money or when she reviews credit card bills with my restaurant deliveries. I don't want to face her, but I have no choice at this point.

I distract myself from reality with a small binge and purge before calling her back.

"Hello?" my mom says.

"Hi, Mommy. How are you?" I would give anything right now to talk about the weather.

"So . . . Kent spoke with Heather. She said you are depressed?" Depressed is not a word in our family's vocabulary.

"Yeah, I am. I just can't do anything . . . my eating is really bad."

My mom has discussed my eating before. Usually, though, her tone is fiery, like spicy jalapenos that make your insides sweat and burn.

"Heather said you needed to go into a rehab." Heather's conversation with Kent must have taken a serious tone because my mother is doing her best to show compassion. I wonder if Heather told them about my suicidal thoughts.

"Yeah, I guess. Everything is just out of control." What an understatement! Things have been out of control since I was sixteen. But the progression has never been at this level.

"She mentioned a place called Sierra Tucson. Do you know how much it costs?" she asks me. "It's around $34,000 for twenty-eight days!" My mom refrained from her usual solution for me. *Greta, at some point, you just have got to get yourself together. You need discipline and structure.* "That's a lot of money, Greta. I don't know if we are going to pay for that. Kent and I will have to talk about it."

Even though I have been through two hospitalizations in Kansas City, we all know that this is unchartered territory. Now my mental health is at stake. I'm sure Heather probably did toss around words like "suicidal ideation" and "keeping her safe."

A few days later and after a couple more conversations with Heather, they decide that they will pay for me to go to Sierra Tucson.

As promised, my roommate Vivian went to her father's house. I only leave the apartment to binge and check the mail. A few days before my scheduled departure, I receive a letter from Sierra Tucson. I open it up. "Admission Information" is at the top, following by a compilation of helpful information in "planning for your treatment experience." Shit. I'm actually going. Up until now, it hadn't set in that I'm leaving the city. I'm leaving my life.

My parents are willing to spend $34,000 so that I can heal. They're taking a chance on my ability to follow through. Thinking back to my past therapies, hospitalizations, and failed efforts, I've fallen in a deep hole. *You're not going to get better. Who are you kidding? It will be a waste of money.*

If I'm not going to get better, then what is the point of living? *Your only choice is to kill yourself.*

I take out my journal and write two notes: One to my parents, the other to Heather.

To Mommy, Daddy, Kent, and Lavada,

I'm sorry I have to be so selfish and do this, but it's the only thing I know to do. I feel like I'm causing too much pain in your lives, as well as my own. I feel so selfish because I know this will cause you terrible pain—and it will give me great relief. I can't live with myself knowing what a liability I am. It may be painful without me in the beginning, but you'll be thankful later, when you no longer have to clean up anymore of my financial messes, you won't have to worry whether I have a job, or if I'm dancing. You won't have to try to fix me or make me be a responsible adult any longer. The only thing that stopped me before from trying to kill myself was thinking about how much I'd miss you. I will miss you. I just think it's best to end things this way. You've been so kind and generous by offering to pay for this hospitalization. And you've always tried to help me any way you

*can. Rather than chance wasting $34,000, I'd rather you
save your money and let me end my suffering.*

*What if this hospitalization doesn't help? I will
just end up killing myself anyway when I fail again. There
are so many things I love about life, but I cannot bear to
keep disappointing you, as well as myself. Please don't blame
yourselves for this. It's not your fault. I'm just not good
enough for this world. I don't know where I'm going, but
it has to be better than the hell I'm experiencing now. I'm
sorry I have to make this choice, but I think it will be better
for everyone. You are very important to me and I will miss
you terribly.*
Goodbye.
I love you, Greta

Dear Heather,

*I'm so sorry I have to do this to you. I'd rather
not, but I don't know how I'll ever survive in this world.
You've been wonderful with me, but the beast has impris-
oned me. I have no hope of me being free ever. I'm so thankful that the last eight months of my life I was able to connect
with you. I'm so grateful for that. If it was my choice, I'd get
to see you everyday. Maybe then I would get better. Maybe
I will now—in spirit, I mean. I feel so sad that I will not
get to talk to you for a while, but I just don't know what
else to do. It would be my fantasy for you to take care of me
and I could come live with you—as if I were a part of your
family—or maybe I could work with you. But that is not
reality. That is a fantasy. Who wants to care for an adult?*

No one, which is why I have to die because I can't take care of myself, and it's no one else's responsibility.

It makes me so sad to think that I will never get to laugh with, talk to, or hug you again. I'm afraid of abandoning you and myself, but what are my options when I don't have a job, money, a place to live, and debts to pay off. Maybe you'll get relief knowing you don't have to worry about me or have to listen to all of my messages or feel powerless anymore. I just don't feel happiness will ever come my way. I will miss you.

Goodbye.

Love, Greta

ACT II